Lessons From The Pimp

The Party Favors Interviews with Dennis Hof

By Joseph Corey III

Josie Alma Press

Raleigh, North Carolina

Joseph Corey III

This book is dedicated to the memory of Dennis Hof who opened the doors to the Moonlite BunnyRanch and invited me inside for quite a few years.

A deep gratitude is given to Sunny Lane and Bailey Paige for being such fine hostesses when I visited the Moonlite BunnyRanch.

This book contains interviews that originally ran in the Party Favors column at QuickStopEntertainment.com

Contact us on Twitter @yourCanadianGF

First Edition

How I Met The Hof

I learned a major thing while doing interviews for NC State's Technician starting in 1985: Rarely did you talk to your subject twice. Whether working for the school paper, various freebie entertainment rags or internet sites; interviews with a major artist was one and done. There were a few exceptions. I conducted three interviews with Mike Mills of R.E.M. during the band's *Fables of the Reconstruction* tour in 1985 and twice met up backstage. A year later when R.E.M. came out with *Life's Rich Pageant*, I was told by the IRS publicist that the band was wanting to be more than a college rock band and were focusing on different publications for their precious interview time. I never approached a subject thinking I'd ask them about something during our next interview. I made sure that I asked the big questions and got at least two answers that weren't going to be given to everyone they spoke with the publicity blitz. I also learned that anytime someone gave you an invitation to do something when they came to town, or you got out there; it wasn't a serious offer (with rare exceptions).

But that all changed when I met Dennis Hof.

I had known about Dennis Hof for a while before we first spoke. The late '90s found the Pimp back in the spotlight as they became the new rock stars before celebrity chefs became the new rock stars. Brent Owens' HBO documentary *Pimps Up, Ho's Down* that took us into the pimpmobiles of such legends as The Bishop "Magic" Don Juan, Pimpin' Ken, King James, Scorpio, Snooky and Mr. Whitefolks. We even got to see a few of them with their stables of ladies battle for the Mack of the Year award. Later the Hughes Brothers gave us *American Pimp* which featured a few of the familiar flashy suited gentlemen of leisure. But it had one big new face with a different direction. While the Bishop and Mr. Whitefolks operated outside the law as they hustled their ladies around major cities, Dennis Hof was legit. Not legit as a pimp, but that he held a legitimate brothel license in Nevada. His Moonlite BunnyRanch outside of Carson City paid taxes. He had a business with a phone number in the Yellow Pages while his peers remained in the shadows.

Back in 1992, *Saturday Night Live* had a sketch called "Sweet Jimmy, the World's Nicest Pimp." Tim Robbins played a pimp who treated his prostitutes with kindness and offered them a profit-sharing plan. Most people forget this sketch since it came right after Sinead O'Connor tore up the picture of the Pope. But seeing Hof next to the unlicensed pimps that weren't into splitting the booty with their girls made me think that he was the real Sweet Jimmy.

Dennis really exploded as a public figure in 2002 when HBO ran *Cathouse* as part of its *American Undercover* series. The show relied on hidden cameras like *Taxicab Confessions* except instead of public transportation; they had the lens tucked inside the BunnyRanch's VIP bedroom. The first time I saw the special, I didn't get to hear it since the VHS tape was screwed up. Thankfully the Closed Captions let me know what was going on as people came to party and pay to get laid. I wrote about the show in my Party Favors column that was being carried by Ken Plume's Tibbysbowl website. I also wrote about the second special and the first season. The series got away from the hidden camera element and explored life in the house. When Ken Plume brought my column over to Kevin Smith's Quickstopentertainment website, I finally had a bit of clout when asking about interview opportunities. People somehow thought I was pals with the director of *Clerks* and *Jersey Girl*. I wasn't going to correct them. One of the opportunities was a chance to chat with Dennis Hof as the second season of the show was coming up. I immediately said yes. The interview went well, and I sent him a link when my column went live. I figured this was our one chance to talk.

A few months later, he contacted me to see if I wanted to talk to him about another episode about to air. Next thing I know, he called me about the *Cathouse The Musical* special. During both interviews he told me that if I ever come out to Nevada, he'd bring me up to the club. I figured that was him being nice. When my wife (at the time) had to work a week in Las Vegas, I called Hof to see if he would let us visit. He was true to his word. He hooked us up so when we arrived in Vegas, we'd grab a plane to Reno, and he had his limo bring us to the BunnyRanch. Hof was a grand host and took us out for a nice dinner with some of the Bunnies and porn star Anna Mills. He made it a fine meal since that night was also our wedding anniversary. What we didn't know was she was pregnant until a week later. So, I became legendary to Hof for being the guy who brought his pregnant wife to the BunnyRanch for our wedding anniversary. The next morning at the brothel, I sat down with Dennis with my video camera, and we recorded a 70-minute interview about his life and work. I have included a transcription of the Hof/Corey Interview along with my subsequent talk with Brooke Taylor, his girlfriend and star prostitute at that time.

Dennis really did open the doors to the BunnyRanch to us. I stayed in a VIP bungalow in the back. There were waffles with the Bunnies in the dining area. I spent a bit of time seeing how the lineups work and how the ladies spent their time between bell rings. It was strange to be on what seemed like a TV set with familiar faces from HBO, but they all had to keep their day job. Bunny Love had to get laid to get paid. The only difference between the show and reality was that director Patti Kaplan wasn't conducting exit interviews with the folks that had just finished partying. Dennis made sure his guests had a good time if they were getting a drink at the bar to recover their strength. As I left the BunnyRanch, I figured that once more I'd never hear from Dennis again. I was wrong.

How wrong? He emailed about looking forward to talking to me about his next project. I wrote back that I hadn't been contacted about interview opportunities. He responded by telling his press agent that I needed to go on the list. I guess Kevin Smith fans were dropping by the BunnyRanch to live the *Zack and Miri Make A Porno* fantasy. I was an important media outlet.

Dennis invited me to his science fiction themed birthday party. This was the coolest birthday party I've ever attended since I ended up hanging out with

Dan Hagerty. I was a big Grizzly Adams fan as a kid, so I was excited when he told me about the fate of his bear co-star. He also told me about the time he hooked up with Phyllis Diller. I think of his story every Thanksgiving since that night. As much as Hof had created an adult Disneyland, I didn't want to be an employee. Turns out Dennis had a rule that he was the only one of the staff that could hook up with the Bunnies. That took the fun out of working at the "Horniest Place On Earth."

Even after all the interviews we'd done, I didn't have a real clue what Dennis Hof did before he bought the BunnyRanch. The only background he had shared was how he planned on buying a Subway sandwich franchise and corporate wouldn't sell him one. He used that money to buy the Moonlight Ranch that became his Moonlite BunnyRanch. He claimed Andy Kaufman was the one who encouraged him to be the new owner since the duo used to frequent the place together. It would have seemed kind of fishy since Kaufman died in 1984 and Hof finally bought the brothel in 1992. But I knew he wasn't lying about their friendship since at the birthday party, I met Bob Zmuda, Andy's old partner in comedy and Tony Clifton. Eventually I learned Dennis' origins story from his autobiography *The Art of the Pimp: One Man's Search for Love, Sex, and Money*. He worked in the Timeshare resort industry. His job was to supervise and inspire the sales staff to sell those "free vacations" to suckers who showed up eager for discount tickets to a theme park. This background detail put everything into perspective as I reviewed our conversations. He wasn't merely Sweet Jimmy, the Nicest Pimp in the World in his approach to the Game. Hof transformed the prostitution world by approaching the transactional occupation as a sexual Timeshare. The Bunnies were both the salespeople and the real estate. They wanted you to buy time inside them. He inspired the Bunnies with the same techniques he used as a supervisor to get his crew ready to sell. And he wanted them to get the customers to upgrade the party. Why get the studio unit when you can buy into a two-bedroom unit and bring the wife and in-laws? He was all about giving the girls lectures on sales negotiations and investment advice. They were constantly reminded of the fortune they could be getting in a few short months if they focus and follow his training and techniques. He gave off the sensation that he used more carrots than sticks to get the Bunnies to keep booking parties. The Bunnies were Independent Contractors who paid to rent a room at the BunnyRanch among other expenses they carried on their account. Dennis was getting paid whether a Bunny was getting laid or not. But he got paid more if they were partying with paying guests. He was constantly teaching them how to increase their earning potential.

I felt during our chats that Hof was giving me lessons on how to juggle the desires of the customers with the needs of the workforce. Not only how to run a brothel if you ever bought a license, but any business. I suggested he write a book called *House Rules: How to Make Your Employees Love Being Treated As Prostitutes*. But that book cover might earn a corporate supervisor a trip to their superior if they brought a copy to work. Once we joked about how he needed to write a business book like the *One Minute Manager* except call it the *One Minute Pimp*. He never did anything on that book since Dennis was going full force with his various ventures. He rarely had a minute. And if he did have that minute, he was going to spend it getting laid.

This book is not an unauthorized biography. *Lessons From The Pimp* are articles and interviews conducted with Dennis Hof while he was alive. He read them and never called up to complain. The only thing he ever demanded I do for him was remind readers that the BunnyRanch was not in Las Vegas. He did get calls from people staying on the strip eager to party only to be shocked that the directions included a 450-mile cab ride.

In Dennis Hof's messages and stories, you should find plenty of lessons on how to manage your workforce. Just do not follow all of them or you will be dealing with the HR Department.

Feb. 20th, 2007

Dennis Hof is America's Pimpmaster General. Over the last five years, he's captivated America by inviting us to get a peek inside his Moonlite BunnyRanch brothel thanks to HBO's *Cathouse*, directed by Patti Kaplan, America's most influential filmmaker. In order to promote the fresh batch of episodes now airing, The Party Favors was given a chance to phone up Dennis Hof, Brooke Taylor and Bunny Love's luxurious hotel suite in Manhattan.

Dennis gave me his history of the show. "It started out in 2002 as an hour documentary under the *America Undercover* umbrella. It was their highest rated non-fiction show. They said, 'Oh my god, let's do it again.' So, in 2003, the same thing. Then in 2005 we came out with the 11-week series that blew the door off all the series numbers. Last night I was with the guys from *The Sopranos* that do the radio show "The Wise Guys." They said, 'Your show equals or beats us OnDemand every week.' Now what we're doing is what (HBO) is calling the second season, I'm calling it the fourth. I don't know who's right. All I know is they've been shooting it for five years.

"You have a documentary, but you also have a soap opera. You got me splitting up with Sunset (Thomas), Me hooking up with the twins. And now me being with Brooke. You have Air Force Amy leaving in a huff. Now she's coming back. You have all this craziness going on in there and it's a business that's operating. And it's a bit of a porn movie. It's everything."

Dennis knows exactly what he's doing in allowing the cameras to probe his life and business.

"My goal in this is twofold. Number one is promotion for my business. I am the P.T. Barnum of Booty. This is what I do to promote my business. And number two: Legalization is the right thing to do. It eliminates all the exploitation. The right wingers like Bill O'Reilly and Sean Hannity will convince you that all working girls are underaged, ethnic, short shorts, crackpipe with a black pimp down the street. They teach you that all prostitutes have diseases and are drug addicts. Why else would they work?"

Prior to *Cathouse*, HBO had aired *Hookers at the Point*, a series of documentaries by Brent Owens about street walkers. It validated the opinions of the right wingers about "the Game" as it was called in Owens' *Pimps Up, Ho's Down.*

"Here we come along," Dennis said. "Oh, wait a minute; look at these girls. They're educated. They're having fun. I told Sean Hannity on camera that these girls aren't working for you at Fox News for 30 years to get a gold watch. They're going to retire in five years with a million-dollar stock portfolio and never work another day. The show changes the stigma. We invited America into our house. And they love our house.

"When I do a conservative radio show, 8 out of 10 people will call in and say "Dennis has got it right." We've got to control this. I look at myself as a guy who is single handedly cleansing this vice. Look at the dirty gangsters during prohibition. Now look at Seagram and Budweiser. Thirty years ago, when I moved to Nevada, it was the dirty little secret of America. The gaming was a dirty secret. Now it's everywhere. The biggest gaming in the world is the California lotto.

"My vision, my dream is to close up half the Starbucks in America and make mini-BunnyRanch Expresses out of them. Stop by for a little tension release. Starbucks has everybody amped up on caffeine. I want to bring 'em down a notch. A guy can come out of his office, go to the BunnyRanch Express and fifteen minutes he's back in his office and it's not so bad of a day for him."

Dennis has seen a lot of changes in the industry in the years since he bought the BunnyRanch. In the first episode of the new season, Brooke Taylor calls her mother after her first party with a paying client. Did the women call back home to share the good news with mom when he first started?

Dennis said, "No. Absolutely not. Fifteen years ago, when I got there, these girls wouldn't tell anybody they were working girls. All that has changed. It's cool to be a Bunny Ranch Girl. (Brooke) called her mom. I've gotten to know her mom. Her mom went on the *Dr. Keith Ablow Show* with her and talked about how they were at Toys 'R Us when (Brooke) told her she was going to be a hooker.

"It's a different world now. I was a very edgy guy 15 years ago. I was a wild cowboy from Carson City Nevada. Now with the internet, (you hear about) all this craziness with dogs, goats and 12-year-olds. And you have the predator series on (*Dateline*) NBC. You've got Bill Clinton trying to prove to the world that a blow job isn't sex. I'm a pretty straight guy, now. I'm a Boy Scout, now. With the sanitizing of this business, has come better girls and better customers. Girls are proud to be here. Guys are proud to say they are customers. It's gotten bigger and better.

While subjects of other reality TV shows control what makes it to the air (Gene Simmons & Hugh

Hefner), Dennis isn't overriding Patti Kaplan's directorial decisions.

"I don't see everything that's on there until the finished product," Dennis declared. "I don't look at the dailies. I don't care to. Whatever it is, it is. I don't give HBO any parameters except to have fun. If something goes on that's crazy or negative, then it goes on. I don't try to control the content in any way shape or form. I don't think it's the fair thing to do for my public. You don't want to make a fluff piece where everything is fine. Did I feel good about Air Force Amy freaking out that time and loading up all her shit? No. I didn't like it at all. But that's what happened. She got herself worked up. She'd been drinking. She's an alcoholic and was back drinking. But now she's back. The sex business is positive. There's a lot of high energy. I don't like negative stuff. But I don't control it."

Dennis enjoyed seeing the first episode of this season since it does feature his new main lady, Brooke getting her start.

Dennis gushed, "That was her first party at the Ranch that we videoed. That was amazing because she looked like a pro pornstar to me. I had to take her to the bedroom and fuck her after watching that."

Of course, the ultimate highlight of the first episode was the introduction of Tiffany, a new BunnyRanch employee who had a strange attitude toward working as a hooker.

"The first show was kinda weird with Tiffany saying, I'm not going to line up. I'm not going to suck a cock. I can't wait to find out what this dumb bitch does in the second show," Dennis said.

Bunny Love at one point had to finish up one of Tiffany's customers since she refused to give a half and half. Bunny was taken back by the newbie's career attitude. "It was an interesting personal choice," Bunny said. "Some girls decide not to do anal. Some girls don't like to do blow jobs."

Dennis chimed in, "Can you believe that?"

Brooke had an even closer encounter with Tiffany when they shared a threesome party. Tiffany however decided that while the customer paid for the attention of two women - only Brooke was going to play. Tiffany reluctantly dropped her top and barely touched the guy on the arms.

"Tiffany is a trip," Brooke said. "I asked Dennis, did she come in just for HBO? I thought she was completely obnoxious." Brooke didn't enjoy sharing a client with Tiffany in the party. "She didn't do anything. From what the producer told me, she acted like the (client) wanted her more. He did not care about her."

Brooke is proof of how Patti Kaplan is the most influential director in America. A few years ago, she was merely a fan of the show. She had a nice job in a nice town in middle America. She decided to step through the screen and be a part of the action.

"How I found out about the Bunny Ranch was from watching *Cathouse*," Brooke said. "I met Carla from the last series when she came back to the Ranch. It was like meeting a celebrity. I'm like, do you know how many times I've masturbated to you? I could quote all her lines. I was a fan of the show so it was really exciting to be a part of it. To hopefully be an inspiration to other girls like they were to me."

While many women get into the business, few have their early days documented. How did Brooke feel knowing that millions of Americans would be following her progress via HBO? "I'm the type of person that if I'm going to do something, I'm going to do it full force. And that's how I took it doing the *Cathouse* series. That's why I told my family. I might as well be honest and go full force with it. Balls out, so to speak."

The episodes were shot nearly a year ago. What does Brooke think when she sees herself arrive at the airport ready to embrace her new career? "I was completely green," Brooke confessed. "I watched the first episode and I see how wide-eyed and innocent I was. Doing the sex scene, I was really nervous beforehand. But once I went in there, you don't see the cameras. I had had sex before numerous times, so it took over and I just had fun with it."

Along with embracing the career, the series documents her becoming Dennis' new girlfriend. She had never been in an open relationship, but as they approach their first anniversary, she seems very comfortable with the dynamic. "Yeah. I view people's sexuality as an individual not as a couple. I completely understand men's urges and desires. If they didn't have those urges and desires, I wouldn't be in business. Having been in this business, it helps me to have a relationship like I have with Dennis. It's nice. I totally appreciate when I can find a hot girl and bring her home with us to share. Sharing is caring."

A major test in the relationship occurs when Sunset Thomas returns to the Ranch to see Dennis. During the first two specials, Sunset was Dennis' woman. Was Brooke nervous at the ex-girlfriend haunting the ranch?

"I was OK with it," Brooke said. "I figured if Dennis had wanted to be back with Sunset, he'd be back with Sunset. HBO kinda wanted controversy, but I hope I didn't give it to them. Sunset was very nice to me when she was there. It was awkward cause I didn't know how she would be and she didn't know how I would be. I think it went OK. My nerves about it came from other people. We knew she was coming in so people kept saying how do you feel about Sunset coming here? Sunset! Sunset! Sunset! Stop relax, it's all OK. And at the end of the day, it all went fine.

"I think if it happened today, I'd have no problem. I wouldn't have any nerves. I'm very secure with Dennis now. It was the beginning of our relationship. We were still getting to know each other. It kinda threw an imbalance in there. But I just stayed with what I knew. I knew that I was with him. I was at the Ranch. She wasn't there. She was coming in to visit. I tried to remain as calm as possible. I think the people around me were more afraid of my reaction to her than I was."

She has grown a lot in the year at the Ranch especially when it comes to exploring her bisexuality. "My first experience with a woman was at the BunnyRanch. Over this year, I've really grown to enjoy them. I'm interested in seeing how my interactions with women are on the show. I know what it is now, but I want to see the differences."

One of the women Brooke was able to please was Isabella Soprano, America's Sweetwhore. "I'm in love with her. She was my favorite from the first show. You'll see me and Isabella doing some things together. We have a little fun together."

Isabella has made a splash starring fetish films and is no longer working at the Ranch. "She came down for the show and worked a bit. She made herself some money and is raising organic vegetables now," Dennis said. "They work and do really well. Then they'll hook up with a guy and the first thing he wants is for her to quit working. As soon as they split up with the guy, they're back. That's what I envision for Isabella."

Another fan favorite to the Ranch is Bridget the Midget. Dennis has good news for her fans. "She had a baby and is coming back to work in the next week or so."

Unlike the first special where the room negotiations were secretly filmed, the clients in the series know about HBO's cameras ahead of time. Only one room in the house is wired up with the hidden cameras. HBO's folks do an amazing *Candid Camera* job to keep out of the way of the real performers in the room. "We don't know where they're located in the room," Brooke said. "They don't tell us where they're at. I kept looking for them and I couldn't find them. I'm glad they didn't tell me where they were because it helps me to forget they are there."

Dennis is in the process of writing a book about his business for Harper Collins. "There's *No Business like Ho Business* was the title Judith Regan liked," Dennis said. He's now considering *Pimp'n Ain't Easy*. I suggested *Pimpin' Made Easy* since people want to buy a book that simplifies the process.

People always like to ask Dennis about the Potter Twins. They were his rebound girlfriends after Sunset Thomas. Dennis has warning for those that dream of such a situation. "The two of them were a handful together. You separated them and they were very normal. You couldn't go to dinner and sit between them. It was like playing ping pong. One would say one word of a sentence with a subject and the other one would pick up a skit from Second City. And they'd go back and forth. It'd make you nuts. They're so bright they're silly. So that didn't work."

So, what is next on Dennis' carnal "to do" list? "Triplets," Dennis said. "I'm like the Fonz. I'm looking for the Hooper triplets. You never saw them on the show. But I'm looking for the Hooper triplets."

Recently the show was visited by FoxNew's Sean Hannity for his *Hannity's America* series. Dennis enjoyed tripping up the self-righteous Hannity by being a perfect host. "He's just a fish out of water there. But he loves the place. He's a man," Dennis said. "He's got Brooke and Bunny in bed. They're wearing scantily clad nighties. He took it in the homes of America at 6:30 on a Sunday night. He stands over the bed and asks the girls "Do you believe in God?" He's waiting for one of those answers that they back into it like "maybe" and then he's going to rip into them. Simultaneously these girls said "No!" It was like game over. He had this deer in the headlights look that was just fucking priceless. He had no idea where to go with that. He just looked at them."

Fans of *Grizzly Adams* were delighted to see Dan Haggerty conducting a wedding at the brothel. It turns out that this is not a one-time thing as another Ranch nuptials is in the works. "We're trying to confirm a date with Dan," Dennis said. "I got him ordained. Dan is the official pastor of the Bunny Ranch." Shame they can't get Bozo the bear to escort the bride down the aisle for an extra fee.

With the success of the show, there's been a lot more visitors to the Ranch. Unlike a TGIFridays that's all about getting the customers in and out, Dennis doesn't enforce a buy or split attitude. There's no time limit to sitting at the bar and meeting the various women that have appeared on the show. "Some guys do come and hang out and don't find anything that they're interested in. Maybe they want to meet every single girl in the whole BunnyRanch before they make their decision," Dennis said. "The guys are very scared coming in there. You watch the show. You go online. You fly out there. The next thing you know, you're faced with a decision of 30 or 40 gorgeous girls. The toughest NFL guy crumbles in front of the girls. 'I gotta get a drink' really means they need a minute to regain their composure."

The question always comes up that on *Cathouse*, guys get charged $5,000 for a fun time. And on Brent Owens' *Hookers at the Point* films, we see guys have sex with skanky street walkers for $50. I ask Dennis if HBO will ever give us a show that allows a guy to have sex without losing the kid's college fund or bringing home an STD for the wife? Where are the clean hookers for the middle-class budget?

"The reality is this, you're going to see a thousand guys spend $200 to $600 at the Bunny Ranch before one guy drops twenty-five grand," Dennis said. "It's better television showing the big parties. That's what HBO does to us. It's almost like you're fishing for whales. We had a guy a couple weeks ago drop $200,000. We had a guy who came in when the first series aired that spent $1.7 million. He never left the place. It's a free market. The girls are negotiable. They're there to make money. Do they want guys to steal any booty from them? No. The guy needs to pay a fair amount. You come to the Ranch, come in there clean, have a good time, make the girls laugh, buy a couple drinks and your money will go a long way in the room.

"Even if you don't want to have sex, partying with these girls is amazing. They're beautiful. They're young. They're vibrant. They're hot. They're skilled. And they're nasty. That's wonderful. Sitting around the ranch having cocktails with 30 girls running around in G-strings - priceless."

It was then that Dennis let me in on a secret. "The guys who spend the big, big money, it's not about sex. Bunny has a guy who spends $30,000 a time, tell him what the party consists of." Bunny continued, "It consists of just hanging out, watching cartoons, going out for dinner and room service. He never watched cartoons before in his life until he met me." There is a man willing to pay $30,000 to watch Adult Swim with Bunny. Dana Snyder is the voice of seduction?

Cathouse The Series is currently airing on HBO. I'm not sure of the time, but it's on around the clock if you have HBO OnDemand. If you're interested in visiting the Bunny Ranch, it's located in Carson City - not Las Vegas. Carson City is about twenty minutes between Tahoe and Reno. Tell Dennis you're a friend of the "Party Favors" and you'll get an extra olive in your drink.

May 11th, 2007

Dennis Hof called the other day to remind me that the next episode of *Cathouse* will be on HBO. "Why They Come" starts airing on Friday (May 12) and hits HBO OnDemand shortly thereafter. "The popularity of the show is so huge that rather than giving an 11-week series, they're giving one show a month," Hof said.

The new installment "interviews couples and guys about why they come to the Bunny Ranch. What's the reason behind it? One of the things that I loved was a ring toss. That's what a guy wanted. They have different sized rings and girls stand back and take aim. The girl that gets it, gets it."

We start discussing how Dr. Ruth once talked about using large onion rings as an erotic ring toss. game. Hof lets me know that the Moonlite Bunny Ranch (in Carson City, Nevada) does cater to the food fetish inclined. He spoke of a regular that enjoys making the Bunny Babes sweeter.

"He will fax us a list and our driver goes down to our local grocery store, Albertsons, and buys about a couple hundred dollars' worth of food," Hof said. "It's always different things. He spends a lot of time coming up with these ideas. Maintenance empties out a room. They put a plastic tarp down and he goes to work. It's all fun and partying. Ice cream, sprinkles and syrups. You name it."

Bunny Love has done food fetish parties with the regular client. "I really appreciate the banana," she purred. "He likes it all. He likes the syrup. Anything that gets really messy." Lobster? I suggest. "Would you pay to eat a lobster off me?" she asked this reporter. "Think of all the butter. You have to have real butter," she demanded. Why did this interview have to be done over the phone? Bunny Love has no idea how nasty and messy I can destroy and pick clean a Maine lobster. Although such a moment would allow Anthony Bourdain to finally have a visual definition of Food Porn. Unfortunately, the food fetish guy isn't ready to step in front of the camera to share his dining tips.

A big note to *Cathouse* director Patti Kaplan: I'll perform the lobster fest on Bunny if HBO picks up the tab. Have a plastic bib, will travel!

How have people been reacting to her appearance on the show? "For the most part, people like me. They think I'm a goofy, buffy, dorky girl. That's alright. I like it." Thanks to the internet, Bunny has been keeping touch with old friends. "A lot of people from high school send me Myspace messages and emails. I was a big tomboy and had a mohawk for a majority of high school. They used to say, 'Why don't you dress like a girl? You'd be so cute.' It wasn't my thing. So now they see me on the show and send me messages saying, 'I was right!'"

One of the big characters this season was Tiffany, the woman who tried to work as a hooker without having to give blow jobs. Bunny has very brief memories of this woman. "She made me look better. I had to handle her business." The episodes were taped over a year ago, but some viewers think the show is nearly live. "I get people all the time saying, 'You should fire that Tiffany girl!' They think she's still working here." Tiffany lasted only two days. Bunny Love will be celebrating her second year at the ranch in July.

The show has made new clients think that the show is always being filmed. "People think we have cameras in our rooms," she said. They're always scoping the scene. They're trying to find out where things are hidden. The only cameras that we have are surveillance for the girls' protection in the hallways. When HBO is there, you know they're there. You're not going to accidentally end up on film."

"Some people want to be on film. I don't know if it's for their 15 seconds of fame or so they can be a porn star and make a little money off it. What's better than coming to the BunnyRanch where you were going to pay for sex and in turn, you're getting paid to have sex?"

The significant difference between Bunny now and when the shows were filmed can be found in her mouth. "I used to wear my retainer all the time so I sounded like a dork."

For those of you folks (like myself), begging for an Isabella Soprano update, she's not working at the Ranch although she is on the series. "She's pretty much retired and hanging out with her vegetables," Bunny reported.

Lately Bunny has been pondering entering the world of adult videos. "I've talked to people about it before. For a long time, I wasn't considering it. But I've been talking to folks in L.A. I'm thinking about seeing what they have to offer. I'm pretty picky. I've got it so well at the Bunny Ranch. It's kinda dumb for me to branch into other areas if it isn't financially worth it."

We discuss the rift between hookers and porn stars. Bunny said., "Some of them are cool with us. There's kind of a beef between porn stars and hookers. Unless you're a contract girl, porn chicks make in one set what we can make in 30 minutes. There's beef there. For the most part I get along with no matter what."

The Bunny Ranch was noted for being a crossover brothel when a few years back it started featuring porn stars as guest hookers. There was a lot of resistance in the porn community over this "meet your fans" opportunity. But quite a few crossed over.

"They love it, too. That's why some porn stars are for it. They see all the money that can be made so they hop on the bandwagon. It's also the same with hookers and strippers. (The Strippers) think they're better. They think we sleep with more people than they do. It's all the same. It's all about money. And we're getting more," Bunny said. "We're giving them satisfaction. We're not giving them visuals."

The success of *Cathouse* was something she saw coming. "I came into the BunnyRanch right after they had finished the first season. I saw all the media attention. You could tell it was going to blow up. It was kind of a bummer that I missed the first season."

The brothel hasn't turned into a place where hopeful actors appear to get facetime on HBO, "I don't think customers are concerned about screen time as much as being a part of the experience. I've never seen anyone adamant about being on camera," Bunny said. "If you act like yourself and have fun, they'll want to film you."

Cathouse is directed by Patti Kaplan. I asked Bunny what it's like to work with the most influential director in America. "Patti is a nice handful. She's fun. She's a kick in the pants." Even though Patti has worked for years making HBO's *Real Sex* series, she's not jaded by filming in the Bunny Ranch. "You can tell sometimes that she gets excited when ideas come up. She says "What!" and you can see her jaw drop. I think she has a good time."

The phone was passed over to Brooke Taylor, the newbie of the show has gone from a semi-innocent girl from Illinois to a queen of the Ranch. How does she react to those episodes showing her arrival in Carson City? "It's kinda like looking at your junior high yearbook. Why did I wear my hair like that? It's fun."

She's been doing more than just working at the Ranch. She seems to pop up in a variety of places with Dennis and Bunny Love. "It's nice to travel and meet all the people. Everybody knows what I'm doing so there's no reason why I can't be open and honest about what I'm doing. I'm having a great time."

Brooke appeared on Sean Hannity's Fox News special "I enjoyed it a lot. I felt I got a couple good digs on him."

One person who had a dig on her was that Tom guy. "I had a Myspace page until it was deleted. I got deleted. They haven't responded to tell me why. I didn't have any nudity," Brooke complained. None of the other Bunny Ranch women had their sites yanked. "The Myspace dude (Tom) is not my friend anymore." You hear that Tom?

Tiffany came up in the conversation. Brooke has finally seen all the footage since our first conversation. She too was taken aback by the blow job-free hooker-wannabe. "I thought she was planted. That's like me saying I want to be a janitor, but I don't want to touch trash. Pick a job that you like the job description. I want to be a stripper, but I don't want to dance."

Stripping is a profession that Brooke had zero interest in pursuing. "There's something about standing there naked and they don't have to pay. Plus, where I'm from, you get a lap dance for a dollar. I don't work for a dollar bill. That's why stripping didn't appeal to me. If they put a dollar on the stage, you have to put your breasts in their face. Not for a dollar."

When I ask about how things are going with her and Hof, she calls out, "Dennis, are we dating?" He says something I can't make out. "Yes," Brooke replies. "We are."

The series shows the relationship developing between Hof and Brooke. "It is our courtship on film. HBO was just out there filming again. It was completely different this time around since I've been with him for a little while now. There's a little more security there then the first time around.

"I was a fan of the show and I was never impressed with Dennis' choices. I always thought he could do better than that. I didn't think Sunset

Thomas treated him well. I thought the twins were just crazy. No girl that he's been with is going to come back and be a threat. If the twins were great, they'd still be around. So would Sunset."

While there's no crossover episode in the works, the gals from *Cathouse* have paid a visit to *The Girls Next Door*. "We were at the Playboy Mansion not too long ago. We met Kendra," Brooke said, "We told her we were doing a new show called *The Girls Next Whore*."

Brooke sees her show as having an advantage over Hef and his trio of girlfriends. "They don't have sex on their show. Sex sells. We got it. They don't. What people do is watch *Girls Next Door* to get the tease of it all. Then they come to us to get the release of it all.

"If we were on the E! channel, we wouldn't be able to show what we are. They push their limits as far as they can. Being on HBO, it's not television, it's HBO. There's not as many boundaries and rules."

After over a year at the Ranch, Brooke is happy about her career choice. "I have the easiest job in the world. I have the job of being myself. People enjoy or they don't. So far, they enjoy it, so I can't complain," Brooke said.

When Hof gets on the phone, we also joke about *The Girls Next Door*. "We look at ourselves as the fulfillment center for *Playboy, Penthouse, Hustler,*

Vivid and *Wicked*. Let them tease them. We'll please them," Hof promised.

Hof's business book for aspiring brothel owners is still in the works. "I really haven't had much time cause of the TV show. HarperCollins wants to do a 4-book deal. I just have to sit down and spend some time on it." A majority of his time lately has been devoted to the show. "HBO is in there 8 or 10 weeks a year and I spend almost as much time promoting it."

Hof is proud that, unlike a recent trend in Reality shows that are secretly scripted, his show doesn't outline the action. "We don't create any drama. Any drama you see is real drama." We speak of the trend of certain shows that are staged. He hates being compared to them.

"It's not reality," Hof declared. "I don't have any editorial control at all. I didn't ask for any. The attorney asked if I wanted it. I said no. HBO, they're the monsters. Let 'em do their deal. Whatever they show they show. I think Brooke had it right; whatever we give 'em, we give 'em. Now I'm smart enough not to explode or go off on somebody during the show. I don't do that anyway in my real life. If there's a situation in the house of something negative, like too much alcohol or drugs with a girl, we're not going to broach it with HBO there with a camera. It's a personal thing with the girl and it's my job to help her with it. We just do our deal and just have fun with it. The ratings are incredible and that's way."

He sees the segments where the girls and clients are learning about new toys and sexual pleasures as vital to the show. "I think education is extremely important. We have shows where they're educating girls and others where I'm talking to guys. There's so much people want to learn about sex. They know so little. So, it's our job to give it to them."

He does have very little to give Deborah Jeane Palfrey, the alleged madam who turned over her customers' phone numbers to ABC news. "She's Madam Scumbag. That's what she is. She's outing her clients. That's the first rule of our business, is privacy and discretion. She broke the cardinal rule. I hope she ends up with the ugliest girl in the penitentiary."

Dennis was recently in the headlines when he had the firemen burn down the Mustang Ranch brothel that he had bought from the government.

"It was the right thing to do. It gave firemen many experiences there that they can't recreate," Hof said. "They had a 20,000 square foot building with eight wings. They got to do a bunch of exercises to see how a fire acts within a building. They controlled the burn. Theory is one thing, but practical experience is priceless. It was the right thing to do."

The burning brothel proved to be a news sensation as Dennis found his name all over the global media. "I was even in the South China Post!" he said. "I did the right thing for the fire department. I got a (tax) write off and I got giant media exposure for being a good guy." He did get a nasty phone call from the former brothel owner who is hiding from the US government in Brazil. "He did call me and said some threatening things to me after it burned down. I said, 'Bring it on.' There's nothing he can do." This ensures that we won't be seeing *Cathouse: The Rio Vacation.*

Remember that each month will bring another episode of *Cathouse* to HBO. If you want to stop watching the show and live the dream, visit www.bunnyranch.com for details.

December 28th, 2007

Why start off the New Year by staring at the skeletal remains of The Crypt Keeper and his son (Dick Clark & Carson Daly) or the skanky duo of Ryan Seacrest and Tila Tequila? HBO is giving you a sexy reason to drop your ball at 12:05 a.m. with *Cathouse: The Musical.*

Dennis Hof has allowed America a peek behind the curtain of his Moonlite BunnyRanch to see how a legal brothel runs. This year he's raising the curtain and putting on a show worthy of a Mickey Rooney-Judy Garland movie. This isn't an amateur hour production.

Who came up with the brilliant idea of a musical that's geared toward heterosexual men? Hof and a few of the Bunnies phoned up the Party Favors to explain this entertainment spectacle. "Sheila Nivens calls me and says, *'Cathouse: The Musical.'* I said,

'Great! Let's do it.' And she said, 'Can you sing?' 'Sing? I banged 11 out of 13 girls in the church choir. Of course, I can sing. Hell ya, I can sing.' 'What about the girls?' 'They can sing, too. If they can't, we'll make 'em sing. We'll teach 'em.' That's what happened."

Nivens picked out a special song from *42nd Street* for Dennis to croon. He was up for the challenge. "They started sending out singing coaches and choreographers to teach the girls and me. We've been in the process of this special for ten months at least."

This wasn't merely having girls lip synch around the BunnyRanch while servicing V.I.P customers. "They really spent the money on this," Dennis declared. "For the filming of the musical, I had them go to Piper's Opera House. It's a historic place in Virginia City. Five or six presidents have been there for events. Mark Twain was in a play there. HBO paid a year's rent on the building. They spent a fortune building all the sets. As much effort has gone into this one show that has gone into the entire 11-week series."

There would be more musical accompaniment than the proverbial piano player in a whorehouse. "We've got a whole band. We have a whole orchestra," Dennis said.

Patti Kaplan, the most influential director in America, tapped into her inner Bob Fosse to capture this spectacular. The hour-long special mixes the women singing and dancing with their everyday work. This isn't just a cut and paste musical performances that you'd catch on PBS during pledge month. Dennis is still amazed at the transitions.

"We used my nightclub as a rehearsal space. The decor is a little bit like the Ranch. When you're watching the rehearsal, it looks like we're in a different part of the Ranch. They filmed all the tryouts; the dance rehearsal and they mixed all this stuff up. You'll be seeing at the Ranch a bunch of girls sitting around a Sybian. Brooke comes out, gets on the Sybian and has this earth-shattering orgasm. It flips into her song. It's a beautiful set and she looks like a million dollars. It's amazing how they led into all this stuff."

Brooke is proud of her song, but can't let her mother see the whole performance. "Right before I do my solo, which I want her to see, I do a sybian ride which I don't want her to see. I told her that she's going to have to close her eyes until that point and she'll just have to guess when to open her eyes. But I lied to her and told her that I faked it so she'll think it isn't real anyhow. There's no way you can have a fake orgasm on a Sybian. It's impossible. They're good for a couple times a year, otherwise I lose feeling."

There were a lot of other non-fake sexual moments captured by the cameras. "It's just an amazing undertaking and it was fun," Dennis said. "Here we are on these sets and the girls are doing their thing. During the breaks they're having sex with each other in the corner. It was like a *Chorus Line* in the *Cathouse.*"

Bunny Love swears she wasn't part of the off-stage hanky panky. "No. I'm gay for pay. So, there wasn't anyone there that I was interested in touching."

During the sound mixing, the head of the post production facility told Dennis that on the average "live concert" by singing superstars they make dozens of pitch tone corrections. "On Brooke's songs they made three," Dennis proudly reported. "They're pushing her to do a pop album."

Brooke was up to the challenge of being in a musical. "I have a degree in music," she said. "It was exciting and then daunting that first came to my mind. It was a lot fun and a lot of work. I did the most songs. I had one day off in the three weeks they were up here filming. That was only because I said, 'I had to have today off.' It was tough. It was a whirlwind. When it was all done, I wish I could gone back and done it all over again."

Was she more nervous seeing this special or the first time she partied with a Bunny Ranch guest? "I have a deep-rooted background in music," Brooke said. "I had to live up to my education and my background. This was more personal for me. I was more nervous about this. Can't I just give a blow job? Can't I just get naked? Isn't there someone I could have sex with?"

Brooke does seem amazed that she's been able to pull off a career move that will set her college career advisors in a tizzy. Has anyone else been able to land an HBO musical special while working at a legal brothel?

"I'm an entertainer," Brooke said. "I'm using all of my oral skills."

This has been a fascinating life for her as she puts her college degree to work. "I've been really lucky to bring in all aspects of my life that I enjoy sex, music, meeting people and traveling," Brooke declared. "People are telling me that I'm exploited in this job, but I'm doing great. I'm doing everything that I want to do and I'm getting everything out of life that I'm putting into it. (The Musical) is one aspect of the job that I never imagined and I'm very thankful for."

She does wish that they could perform the show live. "We'll let you know if we start touring. We'll definitely come to your city," Brooke promised.

Bunny Love wasn't overwhelmed at the concept of the special. "I thought it was pretty amusing of an idea. I'd seen it done before on *Buffy the Vampire Slayer* and *Scrubs*. I thought it was a crazy idea, but if anybody can make it work, we can."

Her background prepared her for the experience. "It wasn't that big of a deal for me," Bunny Love said. "I've done productions with ballet and theater so the lights and the cameras didn't affect me so much. It was just about learning my routines and steps."

Bunny and the others still had to put in hours at the Ranch, but it didn't wear them out. "It's not like I was doing something for a different employer. They understood that you needed rehearsal time and can't be on the floor for your normal shift. It was stressful and tiring, but we pulled through it."

Will the experience lead Bunny Love to appear on *Dancing with the Stars*? "Lord, no," she said.

Air Force Amy was game for performing. "You never say 'no' to anything around here cause you never know what it'll develop into. I said, 'If you want me and think you can do something with it, go ahead. I'll be available.'"

She's been working at the Bunny Ranch for quite a bit of time. How weird was it to realize that she was going to be singing and dancing instead of her normal duties for the show? "It's all weird. It's absolutely hilarious," she said.

During our conversation, we remembered the cinematic joy that was Burt Reynolds and Dolly Parton in *The Best Little Whorehouse in Texas*. "This ain't the first musical to come out of a brothel," she said. Although *Cathouse: The Musical* should be the better of the two.

The only artistic difference that Air Force Amy had with the production came down to footwear. She discarded the shoes provided by the wardrobe mistress. "I brought my own shoes. I'm wearing Chanel. I'm not doing a musical that's going to DVD without wearing my Chanel."

Air Force Amy really did serve in the military. While stationed in the Philippines, she saw Bob Hope's USO show. It's nice to know that troops around the globe will have a little holiday entertainment when she and other bunnies perform "I Know What Boys Want."

I'm saddened to report that Isabella Soprano is not part of the musical. She's still at her organic farm in New England. I was hoping to see her solo with Spinal Tap's "Sex Farm."

Dennis is juiced about the upcoming special. "People are going to be amazed. You expect hooker to suck and fuck and satisfy a man. You don't expect them to be educated, articulate and talented."

He sees this special as altering the way folks will enjoy the New Year after the Time Square ball drops.

"HBO has given us the prime slot. I'm getting hundreds of emails from people saying they're having *Cathouse* parties at their homes. They want us to send them menus. I'm going to spend my whole

New Year's Eve calling various parties and saying hello to people. It used to be Dick Clark from Time Square, now it's Big Dick Daddy from the Bunny Ranch on New Year's Eve on HBO."

Why would anybody want to watch a pack of whores like Carson Daly and Ryan Seacrest when there's a chance to watch the fine ladies of the Bunny Ranch? After a year of having to endure your kids endless viewing of *High School Musical* and *High School Musical 2*, it's time to put them to bed, pop the second bottle of champagne and remember that New Year's Eve is an adult holiday.

Hof/Corey Interview
October 6, 2008

Corey: Can you say something for me?

Hof: Testing 1 2 3 4 5 69 it's mighty fine but I like Oreos.

Corey: Now what is an Oreo?

Hof: Oreos? Well around here around here it's not Oreos. The girls called them Whore-eos. Everything at the BunnyRanch is Ho. Let's go see a Ho! Show. It's a Ho time. It's showtime. Everything is Ho. When a girl goes to another girl's room, because they might be having sex in there, they don't knock. Management knocks. The girls Ho Scratch. They scratch the door with their nails. That way if you're having sex, it really doesn't interfere with you. They're gonna say busy or come on in I need you. One or the other.

Corey: I did not know about the scratch.

Hof: Well, "Ho Scratch" is part of the BunnyRanch vernacular.

Corey: Are there any other words or Bunny vernacular that you think the average person at home would appreciate being able to use in their everyday conversations?

Hof: Well Bunny style is like doggy style except the Bunnies originated and so it's Bunny style. You also have the Freak of the Week party. Every family should have that. You sit down, decide something you haven't done. Let's get a little freaky. Let's raise the bar. Let's be a little silly. That's how you keep your man happy. That's why the Bunnies know how to do these things and typically the civilian chicks don't. These good Bunnies don't say no. Very seldom. I mean all girls have their limits, but the Bunny girls have higher limits and so typically they don't say no. Airforce Amy will tell you that the way to keep your man is don't say no. Even if you don't do what he wants, don't say no. Because once you get into it, a girl can lead the party in any direction she wants it to go. She could make a man have an orgasm pretty much when she wants to.

Corey: After encountering Milla here, pretty much the bar has been raised pretty high.

Hof: Milla, you know Milla the queen of nasty. She takes porn to a whole other level. She won the nasty award every year. Nastiest chick in porn because she does crazy things. I've seen her do an 8-color art piece. It was amazing. By taking a non-toxic paint and putting it inside her and squirting it out all over there. I mean Picasso would be jealous. It's beautiful artwork. I've got one somewhere. I need to put it on the wall out here.

Corey: Do you often get people from the porn world coming over to do guest visits at the place?

Hof: We've been here 16 years and we've had 700 porn girls here. There's three or four here right now. Mila is here. Jasmine is here. We got Anna Mills. There's always three or four. Sunny Lane is coming in next week. Sunset Thomas worked here and lived with me. Teri Weigel. It's some big stars and lots of them that you know. The porn business is drying up a little bit. As that happens, the girls know that they can make money here. They can always make more money here than porn. It's like ten times the money. What porn gives them is some instant notoriety. The parties in L.A. are really not much fun, but they get invited. They feel like a princess because all the fans are there. In here, the fans come to us. The exception is the girls that are part of the blonde squad or the media team that are rolling with me. Then we're at the Emmys and we're at the Grammys and the Billboards and we're backstage at every rock and rap concert. The premiere of movies. We're everywhere. Those girls get giant notoriety.

Corey: Do you feel you're the bookend to Hef (Hugh Hefner of *Playboy* fame) when you show up with your three blondes?

Hof: Absolutely. When we're at the Fox Reality Awards, you got this beautiful stage and the theater and all the tables in the middle. *Survivor* here. P Diddy's girls. Flavor Flav. All the different shows - they're out there and on one side a little orchestra area elevated about three feet up is Hefner and his girls and me and my girls and my bitch Ron Jeremy. We're there and we're like the new image -The new nouveau hip sex people. Not that we're that young but we're younger than Hef. We've got the hot young girls with us and my girls switch up so I've always got different girls with me. And he's got the same three girls. It's nice he's got three girlfriends...three wives if you will. But how could he be with them forever? You know it's like having three new Mercedes and driving the same three the rest of your life. I don't want to do it. I'm glad he can. He's man enough to do it. God bless. But I'm not. (*Editor note: Hefner broke up with his three girlfriends shortly after this interview.*)

Corey: And a big difference is with the three women that you bring to the party; if anybody at home goes," Oh, I'd like to have a chance with her!" Well just come on down to the BunnyRanch.

Hof: That's the beauty of it. When you watch Hef's show (*The Girls Next Door*), you're not gonna have sex with those girls. You may masturbate to their centerfold. That's nice. But I don't like self-service and most people in America don't. Our clients, our friends can watch our TV show, see us at an awards show and say, "Wow. That Air Force Amy is looking really good. I'm going to go to the BunnyRanch." That's what the success of our show is. Finally, these are goals that are attainable for the average man. He doesn't have to just look at the show. It heightens his sexuality and his desire by watching the show and going, "Whoa! You know what? I'm going there." So, it gives him something to think about. Something to plan for. He's got all these things in his mind because sometimes the travel is almost as good as the destination. It's the planning, the thinking about it, the anticipation and all the things that go with going on a trip. It happens to be this is a sex trip...maybe around the world trip with a Bunny.

Corey: How has the show changed your clientele?

Hof: The show has changed my clientele in a lot of ways. Number one: We are the devirginizing center of America. This is where people bring the virgins now. Instead of these guys scrounging around and trying to get some in high school or college and getting the girl pregnant going through all that, the parents say, "No. You need some lessons, son. Remember when we took you to driving school? Remember? You're a good driver now, aren't you? We're going to take you to BunnyRanch sex school and we're going to teach you about girls, so you'll know what to do when you get that beautiful princess in your life." Because if not, it's a terrible experience. She has no experience. He has no experience. That's a recipe for the worst sex in the world and it just won't last long. So, the virgins come here. Couples! We're now seeing an enormous influx of couples because we had the nerve to show that couples really do these kinds of things. Where in the past you know the only thought was "Oh, it was some whacked out swingers somewhere out there doing these things in scroungy places and all that." It's not like that. We showed it. We had the nerve to show it. Lots of couples come in. We had the nerve to show a 60-year-old woman coming in. Her husband couldn't perform any longer and she still had these sexual desires. He told her to come to the BunnyRanch. "Here's the money. Go to the BunnyRanch." We caught her on camera interacting with another girl. These are giant changes, not only in not only in prostitution, but in sexuality in America. We've made it okay. It's okay to bring your virgin here. It's okay for couples to come here because they were always doing threesomes. The wife just didn't know about it. It used to be that the guy would come in and pick Air Force Amy and Bunny Love and have this killer threesome. Now he brings his wife and they have a threesome with one of them and later on they have a threesome with the other one. So that's really changed. We single-handedly made it okay to sell and have sex in America. We change people's ideas a day at a time. Dave Attell, the comedian, said, "BunnyRanch, one person at a time." And it's so true. One person at a time, we win them over. Even if they don't want to participate in what we do, a lot of people don't and that's great. But it's ok for the ones that do want to. Because they'll say, "Wow, this place is cool. If we weren't married, honey, I'd go there." And she's like, "Yeah. If we weren't married, I'd go there." So, the single guy or the married guy that likes to cheat on his old lady or with her permission are like, "It's okay!" They don't look down like, "You bought a hooker?" Those days are done. We don't need that except in the illegal world. When you get into the idiots of the world like Eliot Spitzer, you know the no glove love gov. You know he's transporting girls across state lines. My guess is that she either brought sex equipment or drugs. Her brother's a convicted drug dealer. Why would she have drugs? Well, she could bring drugs on a train or sex toys that they couldn't bring on an airplane cuz they're gonna get searched. The train? They just go, "Okay, yeah, it looks nice. Have a nice day. So that's my guess and I think we're gonna see this guy in prison. *(Editor's Note: the Department of Justice declined to indict Spitzer on the Mann Act in November 2008.)*

Corey: HBO also does the *Hookers At The Point* series. How do you think that reflects upon your show?

Hof: Let's use this: HBO is the food critic. They want to show you the certain Le Cirque in New York, Spago's of Beverly Hills, but they also want to show you the greasy spoon place and McDonald's. You need to see all ends of it. There are guys out there that are bug chasers that intentionally go out with the girls like that. I did a piece with Diane Sawyer, her highest-rated show ever, in Elizabeth, New Jersey. The highest rate of prostitution in America and half the girls are HIV. If guys want to do that well… If we can't convince them to go to a place where the girls are checked properly, have background checks, where they're not going to steal their wallet, they're not gonna have pimps kicking in the door of hotel rooms and you're not gonna be dealing with girls that are all drugged out. They want to go to *Hookers At the Point* and have that experience; have a nice day. But when it blows up, don't call me. They all want to call me. They met a girl, and they'll call me and say, "She stole my Rolex watch and my wallet. I'm in San Francisco. How can you help me?" Well, I could have given you the directions here last week and you came here. "I know you know there's a network and you know all these girls around the country help me." I'm like, "Are you kidding me? How can I help you? You need to bite the bullet. You lost your wallet...you lost your Rolex. Are you gonna call the police and tell them a hooker then I was dealing with an illegal basis, stole stuff for me? You're liable to get arrested. Now when you deal with criminals, criminal things happen to you. It's that simple."

Corey: So, they think there's like a Better Pimp Business Bureau?

Hof: Exactly. What they don't understand is that in the world of Lil Jon, Snoop and all my other buddies in L.A., Nelly and all that, I am a pimp. The Pimp! I'm the man. The reality is reality: I'm not a pimp. I'm a businessman that has a license to do this. The girls and I are partners to operate our business. If the girls do a good job and are good salesmen and they have repeat customers and I keep my expenses in line; I make a reasonable return on my investment like any businessman. So, I don't accept the pimp at all. Unless I'm with Lil Jon and Nelly and the guys then it's okay. Yeah, you're right, I am The Pimp. I'm the pimp. But in their vernacular, pimp is different. If you get a white news executive that says, "Well you're a pimp!" I'm gonna say, "Excuse me? Are you gonna question the morality of the state of Nevada? I think you need to worry about your own city as dirty as it is. Let's worry about New York City where you have the highest rate of syphilis in America. Aren't you proud? You've got drugged out disease-ridden girls everywhere and you don't do anything about it. Don't call me a pimp. Go out and deal with the real pimps. You know what, I'll go with you. Let's do it together." That stops that conversation.

Corey: So, you're more like a really good strip club operator.

Hof: If there is such a thing.

Corey: A pimp's idea is to control the women.

Hof: Totally. Totally control them. They take all the money. They buy the girl a Quarter-Pounder every other day. They want total control of the girl. They isolate them from their friends and family. Typically, it's a drug environment. We're not doing that. We're zero tolerance here. Zero tolerance - that's it. Get caught, you're gone. Goodbye. You want to try reapplying in three or four months, come back and talk to us. Do you want to go to rehab? What do you want to do? You know we're not so naive to think that there's no drugs in the workplace and it's because there's drugs in every workplace in America. Between the police department and the Attorney General's Office, somebody's smoking weed. Somebody's doing prescription pills. The difference is and we deal with it. We don't try to hide it. The image of prostitution in America is under age, ethnic short shorts, street corner, crackpipe and the pimp down the street in the big Cadillac. When you get here, these are business women. We're a microcosm of America. We deal with the same things America deals with. We deal with divorce. We deal with pregnancy. We deal with deadbeat fathers We deal with drugs and alcoholism. In Nevada we deal with gambling. We deal with shopping addictions. I know girls that have four or five hundred thousand dollars for the clothes. I can show you girls who go into the Chanel store. "I love those boots. What color do they come in? Brown, black, beige and chocolate. I love all four." They'll drop $12,000 like that. So, we deal with everything that America deals with except on a smaller basis. As the owner and their friend...because I am the owner, I am the operator...Suzette's a wonderful office wife's help, I am a boyfriend to some girls I'm a brother to some of them, a financial advisor to some of them and a lover to some of them. I'm a lot of things to a lot of girls. But the one thing we are is family. I care about them. They care about me and their business. We all work together for the common goal to have women treated with respect and be proud of what they're doing. I've taken prostitution from guilt and shame to glamour and fame. There's no question about it. No question. From guilt and shame to glamour and fame. My girls are rock stars, some of them. Brooke Taylor has eight pages in *Marie Claire* right now. Twelve pages in *Hustler*, cover and centerfold right now. An hour show on the Women's Entertainment channel right now. *Mike and Juliet* show two weeks ago They called me immediately after the show and said we'd like to use her as a regular. That's how good she is. She has gone from being a Midwest girl with two degrees working as a professional and not able to pay off her college loans to a girl now that a lot of people in America know and like.

Corey: Have you ever found out that a girl working here does have a pimp and he's subleasing her to you?

Hof: Yes. We have found that. They're very quiet. Because as soon as we know the girls here are gonna say, "You have a pimp?"

"Well, he's really my manager."

"What does he do for a living?

"Well, he makes sure I do the right things and I'm at the right places."

"Okay you got a pimp. Why?"

"I got protection."

"You need protection in here? You got the protection of the state of Nevada and the Sheriff's Office. You got Dennis. You're taking all your money and sending it to this guy?"

"Yeah. I send it to him."

"Why? Don't you wanna have things for yourself? Do you have a car?"

"Yeah. We have a new Mercedes."

"Who owns it? Whose name is it in?"

"I don't know."

"So, if you leave him today, you take the Mercedes?"

"I don't think so."

"You need to wise up. Let us show you a different way."

A lot of pimps are smart enough to know not to send girls here or if they do send him here not to let anybody know about

Corey: Who approached who to start shooting the *Cathouse* series?

Hof: We went to Showtime. Showtime liked the idea. But they wanted it to be a scripted show. They gave me all the reasons. "You give us the scenarios. We can do this in L.A. We can build a set. We'll have actors do this. We'll make more money off syndication if it goes."
All these reasons. I'm like, "No. To make this thing work you need me and the girls and our real personalities in this." And selfishly I want the viewers to see my girls on the TV show and have the desire to come to the Ranch. So, they're like, "We don't know. We'll think about it." We went to HBO. HBO said, "We've talked about you for three or four years now. We just don't know what to do. You've done everything. You've been on every TV show. You've done it all."

"No. We haven't done it all."

"Oh yes. We saw this. We saw that."

"Let me give you the scenario: Same shit, different flies. OK? The BunnyRanch changes every day by the new girls that come in. Every month ten, fifteen, twenty new girls rolling in here. New personalities. New things. Different sex. Crazy girls. One girl likes girls. One is gay for pay. All these different things. That's what's going to change it. We'll have a core group of people that are a permanent part of the show. We'll rotate other people in and out. One girl is going to be extremely successful, goodbye I made my money. Another girl is going to be miserable. Her boyfriend is dragging her out of there. It was his idea and then the reality that she was sleeping with different men and he couldn't deal with it. The girls get mad and leave. Same girls come back. That's what's going to make it all work."

And that's been the success of it. The show is a lot of things. It started out being a documentary. Then we added some sex to it. A little more sex. Softcore porn. Now it's turning into a reality show. It's a docudrama now. It's a soap opera...*As The Bunnies Turn*. And that's what people like. That's what they want because they never know what's going to happen. What the hell? Is Dennis not with the *Penthouse* Pet? He's with these twins. Twins? Who does that? I do. I'm looking for triplets now. I'm with Brooke (Taylor). And Suzette is doing different things. One girl gave her a hard time.

She's gone. Other girls are here showing her a good time. We're having sex education. We're having a class out here teaching girls how to give head. We've seen things this season, fifteen girls sitting around the parlor on their laptops. Because that's the way it is. They're communicating with people. A lot of our business is done on the internet. It always changes. It's always something new. It's always fun and there's no business like Ho Business.

Corey: It seems like a lot of the new women working here are fans of the show. What percentage of the women who come here because the show spoke to them?

Hof: More and more. More, more and more. More people are applying. Over a thousand girls a month go on the internet to BunnyRanch.com, press *Be A Bunny* and apply. I knocked out forty to fifty today before I came here. I'll be getting 25, 30 calls today. As the economy gets worse, there's more of that. Economy is bad. Tough times. We don't feel that recession. There is no recession here. I had a sales meeting a couple months ago and (I said), "Gas is a problem. It's pushing $5 a gallon. A lot of people aren't going to come to Nevada. The news: Tourism down, gaming revenues off." The girls are starting to feel it. We're a sales team. A sales team has to be motivated, excited and believe in their product. It's my job to motivate these girls and keep them excited. Their attitude is getting down. (They ask,)

"What's it going to be like? Nobody is going to come to Reno or Lake Tahoe anymore." So, I do the sales meeting. "Look, Nevada is basically recession proof. This is the worst I've ever seen it in Nevada. But our numbers aren't changing. Here's what's going to happen: You're going to work your customer base harder; you're going to get on the internet and work our message board which has 25,000 - 30,000 people posting. That's what you're going to do. You're going to be available for media when they come in here. You're going to wake up and do radio shows with me at 4 o'clock on the East Coast. What am I going to do? I'm going to think of incentives. Giving away gas cards to customers that come here. I'm going to deal with the media. I'm going to pull the stops out. I'm on the move now. You're going to be seeing less of me because I'm going to be in New York. I've been there three times in 19 days now. It's a brutal trip. I'm going to do my deal. I'm going to put the word out there: BunnyRanch! BunnyRanch! BunnyRanch!" I'm going to look for every angle. Oops, here's one: George Bush stimulus program. You know what? I put the press release out: The BunnyRanch - George Bush Stimulus Plan. After Fifty-Three years of the BunnyRanch providing quality stimulus to America, we've decided to support George Bush who we don't like. When you bring your stimulus check in here - your six-hundred-dollar check - we double the value of the check. We give you a $1,200 party and we're going to have a special: Three Bunnies -

one bottle of champagne - George Bush party. If George was here, he'd be drunk, obviously. We want to do that. We're going to have a big card here. And every guy that cashes his stimulus check here is going to get to sign it. And the Bunny is going to sign below him and say what they did in the party. After the first hundred parties, we're sending it to George. He can't be here. He's too busy fucking up our country. But we're going to send it to George anyway. Huge hit. One hundred and forty television stations around the country picked up on it. American Airlines comes out, "We're going to charge 15 dollars to check your bag." We do the press release: BunnyRanch doesn't like American's program. Our customers like to come and bring their costumes, their dresses, their sex toys and they need to check their bags. And they need to pay $15? From now on, when you pay that $15, get a receipt, bring it to the BunnyRanch and when you bag a Bunny, we'll apply that fifteen bucks to it. These are the things we do. Gas? Gas is not a problem. (I said,) "Girls, it's not going to be a problem. Our customers have money. To show you it's not going to be a problem, I'm leaving here. You know what I'm doing? I'm going to Mercedes and buy a V-12 twin turbo 600 horsepower sedan that gets zero miles to the gallon. I don't care what gas costs! Because we're going to make enough money that it's not going to be a problem." I walked out that door. Went to the Mercedes (dealership). Three hours later I'm back here with the car. "See girls!" And the girls are like, "There's no problem! There's no problem." If they don't think there's a problem, there won't be a problem. Our business is up twenty percent this year. Twenty percent in a time when everyone's business is down. Ours is up twenty percent. Why? Attitude. Attitude isn't important. It's everything.

Corey: Do you think that part of why your business is doing better than the other ones is ultimately you're providing satisfaction. You're giving a moment of "This is a good life."

Hof: This is a good life. I'm the man. Come live my life. Be with me for a day. Get away from all the problems at work. Your business being off. Your wife ragging on you because she doesn't have the money for the shopping she wants. Come in here. Come with me. Hang out. Bring the wife if she's hip. Have a good time. We're providing a service. It's real. The strip club? From the minute you get out of the car to the minute you get in the car, they're conning you. They're leading you to the next step. If you pay twenty dollars, you're going to get to see some titties. Here's twenty dollars. You walk in and you order a drink. In New York recently a bottle of water was fifteen dollars. I didn't pay for it since they comped everything. So, you go in there and order a round of drinks and you're in this 150...200 dollars. The girl says, "I'll give you a lapdance." Lapdance is $20. "Come on, let's do something." Now you spent another $500. You dropped a grand and nobody's gotten laid. Only thing you walk out of there with is a hardon. This is real. Nobody is conning anybody here. The girls have some time. The guys have some money. Everybody is here to get along and have a good time. It's very real. And because it's real, we lose four or five girls a year to relationships.

Corey: Comparing this place to a strip club again; you don't feel muscle when you walk into the place.

Hof: Well, there's no comparison to a strip club with the BunnyRanch. You're gonna get pushed and pulled in a lot of different directions in a strip club. Here? They're just going to pay attention to you. And if you want to do something, you do it. Now what I want is an environment where a guy can walk in the front door, see 20 to 40 girls and be overwhelmed. Like "Oh my god! Oh my god! Do I deserve this? Can I afford this? Is my wife gonna catch me? Am I gonna want to come back here every day? Should I even be here?" That's what I want. Then they either pick a girl or they go to the bar. When you get to the bar, it's the world's best singles bar. The odds are very good. That's what I want. Now if you decide you want to talk to a girl then you talk to her. We let him know all the girls want to talk to you. But we're not going to go out of our way to pressure you to do anything. This is your decision and the guys know that. So, they come in here. They'll have a drink. They'll relax. I'll talk to him. It's casual. In a strip club, they're fighting. It's like 200 girls fighting over a pie for Thanksgiving. Here, there's money for everybody. If you wanna make money, you make money. It's that simple.

Corey: When I said muscle, I meant security guards. When you go to a strip club, there's that feeling that they're out there to break my fingers. They're not happy until my head hits the door.

Hof: Well, they're right. The way the sheriff in Nevada explained it to me when I bought the place 16 years ago was, "If you have a tough security, you will need it because they have to justify their job." The guy is in the parlor; he's drunk and he says something stupid which is what all people do when they're drunk. "Come here, you little whore!" A security guy's gonna say, "Excuse me, Butthead. We don't say whore here!" There's gonna be a fight because the guy, even though he's drunk and the security guard's twice his size, he's got to prove to these girls that he's a man. Before you know it, the security guard is beating the crap out of the guy. That's the strip club mentality. BunnyRanch mentality is the cashier or sales manager goes and talks to him, "There's no whores here. If there's any whores, it's your mama and she's not here. Okay? So why don't you just calm down. I don't want the police to come and arrest you. I'll feel bad they put handcuffs on you because you're in Nevada. Where are you from? California. You're gonna have to see the judge. You can't bond out. Would you be calling your mom or your boss or your minister? Who would you call and explain to him that you were a dick at a cathouse? Who'd you do that to? Let me buy you an espresso. Get a couple espressos going. You know what? It's okay." Now if something happens, we're prepared for it. But you don't you don't see any visual signs of things. We got male drivers. We have a male bartender. But the instruction is unless a guy puts his hands on a girl, stay out of it. Let the women deal with it. If a guy's being smart to a girl, two or three girls are gonna say, "Hey! What's wrong with you? you really need to get laid, don'tcha you. Come on. Let's get a room. Let's get out of here." And that's the end of it. Knock on wood...knock on my hardon, we don't have any problems.

Corey: How much down time and waiting is there for the women who work here?

Hof: The hardest part of this job is waiting. That's why we have so much going on here. We have a gym and a trainer. We bring in chiropractors. We bring in dermatologists. Tune-ups. Waxing people. We have bicycles and ATVs. We're building a bigger gym. There's always something new. We're encouraging all the girls to have a laptop because that's money. That's mining gold. You're typing for cash to get customers to come in here. But it is the hardest part of the job. The hardest part of the job is being away from home and the downtime. That's the hardest part of being a worker at the BunnyRanch.

Corey: Some women have talked about working at other places where they had lockdowns. Once you started your designation shift, you couldn't leave the place no matter what.

Hof: Lockdown, yes. It's very common in Nevada. Most places have it. It's not a designated shift. It's the time that you're gonna be there. If you come in, they want you to stay three weeks. We don't have any minimum or maximum stay. We're like a hotel; once you've been here. The first time you're here, we like to see a girl spend nine days here. They get in on a Thursday, that's when all the new girls come in, that way we can train them in a group on Thursday and Friday. We want them to work that weekend and the following weekend. They leave on Sunday or Monday so they're here for nine days. That we do want. After that "Hi, I'd like to work from the 12th to the 14th?" "Yeah. Well, let me see if we got a room. Yeah. We got a room. You're booked in." It's like a hotel. It's always gonna be a room for them if they do the right thing. If you call and say, "I want to be another 12th and I'll be there for ten days" and on the 12th you're like "my dog ate my pumps, and I can't find my car keys and I missed my flight" - that's a problem. You want these people to be responsible. We've got a hotel. A small hotel and we want every room filled every day. So, if you're responsible and do the right thing, you'll always have a room. If you're not...if you do it once, we're gonna talk to you about it. You do it twice; then the rule is fly up here, go to the doctor and we'll see what we can do. If we don't have a room, be prepared for a hotel. The second we get a room; we'll get you in here. Or you can (stay at) the hotel, come in here and work and then go back to the hotel. But we're not gonna block a room for you because you're not responsible and we don't know for sure you're gonna be here so we're not gonna block a room until we actually see the whites of your eyes.

Corey: How many people working are commuters and not living in the Reno area?

Hof: Probably 70% flying in from all over America and some from out of the country that have proper work permits. They come in to work from all over the United States. You name a city and I'll tell you the girl that lives there. From all over the United States, they come in here. They come here for two reasons. What I share with girls is this: If you don't want to make a lot of money, you only want to make three...four...five...six grand a month get in here and get it done and get out of here. That will take care of you and your children...a lot of girls are single moms with no support from the spouse. Get the money. Go home. They come back next month and do the same thing. The other thing is and it's good for people that are trying to accomplish some goals. They want to be an actor. They want to be a singer. They're working to be Miss America or a fitness program or whatever they're doing. Get in here for a short time, make good money and go. The other thing is if a girl wants to be wealthy, she needs to focus. We've got girls making up to a half a million dollars a year. You got to focus. You got to be here. The longer you're here, the more you're here, the more money you make. It's really that simple. If you want to make a career out of this: Come in here and put in three...four...five years and leave with a million...two-million-dollar stock portfolio or real estate investments. You're set up for life. You'll never work another day. Now is that the reality? No! Because girls have boyfriends, and they give their money. They gamble. They shop. They raise their lifestyle so high. They're driving new Ferraris and they live in multimillion-dollar homes, so they have to keep working. But a girl can work three to five years and never work another day in their life. There's good and bad in all employment, okay. I'm sure Starbucks is fun. But also, people burn their hands there and things happen. The problem with this business as the problem in any business is this: If you go from working as an administrative assistant for twenty-five...thirty-five thousand dollars a year and you come here and you just do okay...you make one hundred fifty thousand: How are you gonna go back to that job? You're not. The second you meet a guy and sometimes they meet him right here and they're such hypocrites. "I don't want you to do this anymore." That's what every girl wants to hear. "I want to be special with you. I don't want you to be with anybody else." The easiest way to get a girl is to tell her you want to be exclusive with her. What are you gonna do? You used to make all this money and all of a sudden, it's cut off because you're in love. He's the guy that doesn't make a lot of money. Once you go through your savings, you get frustrated and you're miserable. The relationship doesn't work. So, come up with your plan. Are you gonna continue your education? Are you gonna save money and get into a small business or are you gonna work hard for a few years and get enough to where you don't ever have to work? Do something. You gotta have a plan? That's a problem to take your girl out of here after making all this money and to put her back into that. We had one girl making $200 a week before taxes at Domino's (Pizza), came in here and made $40,000 in the first month. How is she going back to Domino's? It's never gonna happen. Second thing: I've worked for 16 years and been public about this; I am the first person in this business to go public and be able to tell you why it should be here and why it should exist and put the positive spin on things and deal with the negatives. There's always gonna be a stigma against certain groups. Like in Nevada, you go right into a Bank of America.

"I want to buy a house!"

"What do you do?

"I work at the BunnyRanch."

"Oh Great. You'll have the money to pay."

It's easy. It's acceptable. In certain narrow-minded groups, more or less in religious areas you're always going to be a slut. That's it. They have to be able to overcome that stigma, be able to hold their head high and say, "No. I'm not. I'm a businesswoman. I don't do anything illegal and just because your morals don't coincide with my morals, I'm sorry. The morals of the state of Nevada allow gaming 24 hours a day, liquor 24 hours a day and sex for sale in certain places. Maybe you should worry about your town. We got our problems here. You should worry about that." So, you deal with stigma and you gotta have an exit plan. That's the only problem that I've ever seen.

Corey: A couple of the women I talked to mentioned when they had to come out to their folks about their job, they showed them HBO's *Cathouse*. Their parents didn't think it was that bad.

Hof: Exactly. You're absolutely right about the TV show. We've opened our doors to our house...our cathouse and we've allowed America to come in and spend a little time here. The majority of them like it. Giant ratings from people watching the show. That's really one of the ways. The girls will say. "Watch the show!" and the parents will say, "That doesn't seem so bad. I mean you don't have to do anything you don't want to? You don't have to do anybody you don't want to? You have to do anything sexually you don't want to?"

"No."

"You don't have you don't have to party with a seven-foot 900-pound stinking man? You don't have to do it for any less money than you think it's worth it? Seems to me that's kind of like a singles bar in there."

"Yeah, it's exactly what it is."

The show has definitely changed the perception of the business and gave more credibility to the girls. Because when you don't know about something and you see these horrifying images which the moralist right wing has set up as being this awful destructive drug ridden criminal organized business, parents would have a concern. Once they see (the show), "That doesn't seem so bad. You know what? When I was in college, I would have done that too."

Corey: If the parent only sees the NBC Undercover Human Trafficking Special, they always seem to run every six months, I can understand them being shocked. Do you think it's important on your show that you have money conversations during the staff meetings?

Hof: We bring in investment people. We bring in tax attorneys. We teach these girls how to structure their lives. Probably half the girls here have corporations and financial advisers and stock portfolios. Yeah, it's absolutely perfect. That's what makes a professional business. This is the only business that I know that a girl can not only earn equal money to a Man, but a lot more. It's still the reality of any job a woman has in America, a man makes thirty percent more. So, if he's making 100, she's making 70. That's reality. People say "Aw it's not like that." Bullshit. It is like that and this is the only business that changes. Because excepting in a gay environment; there's no desire for a man to sell anything. It seems unfair cuz I'm like "I'd like to sell something." I'd like to have girls lining up wanting to party with me. In fact, I do except I don't get paid for it.

Corey: When did you become the stud? When did you walk into a room and you know "I can do what I want at this point because when I ask, they will say yes"?

Hof: When I bought the place, I was with a young girl for five years and so I didn't do anything. But when I started doing a lot of television and a lot of radio; I started becoming known and I've got civilian girls asking me to sleep with them instead of me begging like all men typically have to do then the lights went off. "Whoa! I like this. I like this power. This is great. The power for a man to say, "No." How many men in America could get that many opportunities where they can say, "No." They jump on every opportunity they get typically unless there's some situation where they have a girl they're committed to or they don't feel right about it. But men never get enough. When I got to the point where I'm getting civilian girls wanting to party with me, but I don't want to party with them; that's when the lights went on and said, "I am the man. I am the man." Now I've carried this a step farther since the TV show is so popular. There're so many people out there, I don't party with civilian girls. It's like no civilians. I'll have a picture of a civilian girl with a big red mark around it like this (makes a slash in the air). I don't want I don't want any part of it. They don't know about sex. They don't know what to do. They're not gonna please me. No matter how hard they try, it just isn't gonna happen. If you and I are building a racecar, we're not gonna go to the New York school of driving to get some whacked-out immigrant to drive our car. It's not gonna happen. We're going for the driver that ran a thousand races, that's won Indianapolis, been a Formula One guy. That's the guy we're looking for. The professional that knows what to do, that knows how to handle the equipment, that knows every situation that's going to happen. He knows how to deal with it and take a negative and turn it into a positive. If I hear one more guy tell me, "I'm with a girl that's a virgin. I'm with a girl that was only with two guys," I'm gonna puke. Because what that tells me is dude you got bum lay on your hands. Unless you are the man and you had a lot of experience and you could teach her and work her through the steps to get her to the next level: you're going to have a miserable sex life you'll end up in the divorce.

Corey: Unless she escaped from the convent.

Hof: Exactly. Or you come here. You have the wife that you care about and love and she's your friend and the mother of your children. You come here for you to work out your kinks.

Corey: Do you feel you are a target for law enforcement because you are so visible? You were talking the other day about how the TSA just loves to search your stuff. How careful do you have to be when you go to New York City?

Hof: When I'm in New York City, I'm getting police escorts. They love me. I don't think I'm a target. I've never been targeted by anybody. But what I tend to do is make sure I'm not with the wrong people. I don't want to be involved with anybody that's got any affiliation. Even if it's a rapper with gangs or drugs. I don't want to have dinner with anybody that could potentially be a syndicate, Mafia or corrupt person. I associate with a crowd of people, but I can't be with anybody that's got problems. I went through an FBI inspection of my life; it gets updated every year. If I get any problems, I don't own this place. It's really that simple. I'll go so far out of my way that years ago I had a girl that was dating that loved to smoke weed. The first thing I told her was "No smoking here. This is my business. You smoke it at your house, the hotel, or my house. I'm not going to smoke weed. She wanted me to try it so much. I was living with the girl so we flew to Amsterdam. In fact, I took Joey Buttafuoco and his now-wife with me. We went all over there and experimented with it. No big deal. I don't drink. I don't do any drugs. But it was fun. I had fun. But it was legal so if anybody ever asked me. "Do you smoke weed?" "Yeah, I did. We went to Amsterdam once and tried it. I'm not a hypocrite. I'm not going to lie. But I don't have any part of it here at all. It's illegal. I can't do illegal things. (*Editor's Note: Recreational Marijuana usage became legal in Nevada on February 6, 2021.*)

Corey: Is it weird, especially in America, when you see the high-profile busts of madams and pimps; yet you sit back and go "I'm living the life. I'm keeping my nose clean. I'm paying my taxes." Its location, location, location.

Hof: Yes.

Corey: How do you feel when you hear about these people getting busted?

Hof: You really have mixed emotions because Heidi Fleiss, my ex-lover, good friend; she goes to a penitentiary. I'm an hour...53-minute flight away from her on Southwest airlines. I'm going to the governor's ball. It's so moronic that it can be like that. A fifty-three-minute flight away to go to a penitentiary and here you go everywhere. It's really kind of crazy. I see the DC Madame. I see all these people going upside down and I have all these problems. On the one hand, I look out and say damn this is wrong. The other hand I'm like "Dude, you know what you get yourself in for. You knew that you were pimping the pantry. You knew what you were doing so what's the complaint? Do the time. Get it done with.

Corey: What projects are coming up for you?

Hof: The things that are coming up for us are exciting. We've done three shows this year. We did the New Year's Eve musical. We did a Valentine's show and an April show. Now in October, November and December we're coming up with more shows. And they're over the top with fun things. Great show. We're really excited about it. The new things that are coming up with our new shows in October...November...December, we're raising the bar. Hooker Box Office at its best. They're gonna be great shows. Simultaneously, after our first show, two days later, a three DVD box set with season 1, season 2 and the musical arrives. That's exciting to me because now we're gonna be able to get that stuff to the military guys. We'll send a thousand of them to the military guys. People around the world will be able to see it. Outside of America there's not a lot of on-demand. I get emails every day. "How do I see your show? Where can I buy this? So, there's gonna be a huge demand for this product. I see a lot of sales. They're gonna buy it and be able to show it at home. People will be able to use it in their bedroom instead of watching porn they'll be watching Cathouse. It's a softer way to get into the sexual side of things. If a couple's watching this, they're gonna have some sex education in most any show. "Let's try that. Let's find the G-Spot." The nice thing about it is now people will be able to get these things and watch them at home. Guys can watch them with their girlfriends and lead into it. It's like porn light. It's got some softcore stuff, but great sex. It leaves a little bit to the imagination. It allows people to explore. It allows them to talk about threesomes, to talk about anal, for the girls to learn how to give oral by watching watch our girls do it and just have fun with sex. Make sex fun. That's what we're about. Let's make it fun. Everybody's doing it. Nobody wants to talk about it. Let's bring it out in the open. Let's talk about it. Because when our show airs, everybody around the water coolers of America is talking about the next day.

Corey: Now what do you what do you see is the new trend in in sex as far as what people are exploring more now than five years ago?

Hof: What do I see is new trends in sex? The new millennium sex is a less penetration and more fantasy and fetish. You see a lot of that stuff. The guys that are into the foot fetishes, trampling, S&M... all those things. The multitude of them. Kissing...smoking. It's endless. Whatever the baby boomers do then that's the bulge of America. That's where the most sales of a product come from. What the baby boomers do. The baby boomers aren't having as much sex. They're having more fun. They're having more fantasy, more fetish and doing crazy things. Where they used to be able to knock down two or three or four girls in a day. Now it's one and some Viagra for the second one. So, they're not coming in here and partying with five or six girls in a night. That's what the baby boomers are doing. I see guys go up to the bar and the girls go, "Hi honey, let's go party. "I need a little time. I need a glass of water." Slams down the Viagra honey. "You know what? In an hour I'm gonna be hard as Chinese arithmetic." You know Viagra is like Disney. It's a one-hour wait for an eight second ride. "I'm gonna have some fun. Give me a little time." They're open about it. They're honest about it. That's what I'm seeing as the change. I'm also seeing a lot more couples and a lot more virgins which is great for us. I kind of relate it to the Joe Camel thing. You start them out young. Instead of getting laid in the backseat of a Toyota; banging a chick, losing your virginity, getting her pregnant and ruining your life; now, they're coming here when they're young and they come back. They understand instantly the reason for the BunnyRanch. I don't have to lie, because girls want you to lie. "If we do this, you're not gonna do it with anybody else are you?" We all lie. Of course, we're gonna lie. "Just me and you baby." "If we do this, I'm gonna be your girlfriend." "Yeah. Of course, you are." The guy doesn't want a girlfriend. He wants to get laid. They want to get laid. That's what guys want. When they come here for the first experience then they go out and start dating and they start learning things. They come back here and learn more about technique and skills. They get better at it and better at it. They finally realize, "You know what? My job is more important than me sitting around discos until three in the morning and dragging some girl home and getting drunk with her and having to beg her for a handjob." They can come here. If your time means anything, the BunnyRanch makes sense.

Corey: The BunnyRanch is five thousand feet above sea level. How's that affect a guy sexually? For those who visit not from the local area; do guys talk about the oxygen level?

Hof: Some guys are like "Man, I didn't have this much strength as I normally have. But that's a good idea. You come here and train. I'm setting up a boxing camp for Butterbean so he could train in the high altitude real soon. Guys could come here and train to have sex in higher altitude just in case they they go to Mexico City or Colorado or something. They'll be ready for the big game...the big orgasm.

Corey: Butterbean is coming here?

Hof: Yeah. Good guy. He's gonna use this as his training camp. BunnyRanch training camp. We got to get more food.

Corey: You're going to need a bigger kitchen for him.

Hof: We get Butterbean and Ron Jeremy here on the same day; there won't be enough food. That will be the fight to see who gets the last porkchop.

Corey: Are there any celebrity porn tapes that you've watched and said, "Oh God, that's horrible."

Hof: I've never seen one. I know Kim (Kardashian). Not real well. I've been around her many times. She's very close with Joe Francis (creator of *Girls Gone Wild* videotapes). Joe Francis is very close with me. So, we're in the same social setting and done things. Never seen it. Never seen the Paris (Hilton) tape. Joey Buttafuoco's my good friend and I've promoted his tape. I did a lot of marketing to help him. Never seen it. I don't watch porn. I make porn without cameras. I'm the guy that's in the room directing the scene with two or three girls and having a good time. I don't need a camera. I've got it right here. (Points at his head.) This is my camera. I've got memories.

Corey: You're a live theater person.

Hof: Yeah. I'm a hands-on guy.

Corey: Can you talk about all the changes that you've done here over the past three years?

Hof: We're always making changes. It's a constant construction and remodeling project. We have a team of people. We have carpenters, painters, drywall people and wallpaper people. They start at one end of the house and go to the other end of the house and then they go to the other house. Then they start at the beginning. It's constant. In the wintertime, we're working on the rooms. We're repainting them and putting in new furniture. In the summertime, it's the grounds and the exterior to make it more beautiful. We're putting in a new road. We worked for years to get the permits from the state government to put a new approach off of Highway 50. We're gonna have our own road: BunnyRanch Boulevard. (Editor's Note: the street was built, but the address of the BunnyRanch appears to still be 69 Moonlight Rd.) We're gonna name all the streets in here because we're building an industrial complex. Madam Suzette's Way. Air Force Amy Highway. All the working girls are gonna have their own roads in here. (Editor's Note: As of 2021, there seems to be no additional roads with names of the star working girls on the property.) That's exciting to us. We're working hard on an industrial park. We thought, "Let's build an industrial park and have 500 or 800 employees around us. They can come over here at lunchtime.

Corey: If you watch the show on HBO, you get a weird feeling that this place is right in the middle of an industrial auto repair center. Not realizing it's actually just next to it. This road visually will make people see this place is much nicer.

Hof: Absolutely. You're gonna see a beautiful tree-lined landscape well-lit Parkway to get in here. It's gonna change the appearance. Last year we spent a million dollars on the exterior, built a new entry and put in handicapped ramps. We put in ADA approved bathrooms to bring it up to new world standards. The whole exterior is brand new. The parking lot is brand new. We need the approach to get here so you can see a beautiful lighted, well landscaped road to come here. We're gonna have billboards along the way with the top hooker of the month. We'll have HBO billboards.

Corey: You built a gift shop?

Hof: We built a gift shop.

Corey: Did you have a gift shop before?

Hof: We always sold t-shirts, but we never had a place to do it. Now we have t-shirts, water bottles, dog tags, Humping Bunnies Pins… You name it, we got it. We sell a lot of it. It gives people a reason to come in here. They can come to the gift shop and you know they'll buy some t-shirts. They'll come in and say, "Oh I just want to buy some t-shirts." They'll buy some t-shirts, but will be looking in here. "Can I go in there?" "Sure. You want a Coke or a cup of coffee?" "Yeah. I'd like to do that." The next thing you know they're off to the room. They need an excuse to come in here. They got one now: The gift shop. Ten to fifteen years ago, a couple would come in here. It really was an excuse for the girl to get down with a girl. They'd come in here, they pick a girl, they go to the room and they negotiate the party. When the party would start, the girls are getting their clothes off and the guy would say, "You know what, I'm gonna go get a beer. I'll be right back." He would never come back. He wasn't the husband. He wasn't a boyfriend. He was the support mechanism; the reason they came to the BunnyRanch. Cuz it's okay for him. She doesn't know that it's okay for her. She's in there getting down with a girl. Now women executives come in here and say, "You...you...you...we're gonna all go out to dinner and we're gonna come back here and have an orgy." They're more open about it. They don't need an excuse. The gift shop is a great excuse. A $20 t-shirt all of a sudden turns into a three-girl orgy.

Corey: That's a bang for your buck on that property.

Hof: I like it.

Corey: You've got the place across the street. How does that operate?

Hof: We have a place across the street. It's been here 53 years. That one's been here since 1979. It was originally Kitty's Cathouse and then we changed it to BunnyRanch Two. It was just too much confusion, just really too much confusion. It didn't work like we thought it would work. So, we've changed it now to The Love Ranch. It's a Western theme with new management there. We started anew. I've taken the company policies and turned it into a manual and gave the manual to a good friend of mine, Rich. "Here you go, run it like you want it." It's an entirely different operation because Suzette has one way of doing things and Rich has another way of doing things. But they all get it done. Sales are up. The girls are prettier. Some really beautiful girls...and truthfully, I enjoy going over there more. Not intentionally, but it used to be the stepchild. Now it's not that. Now it's its own identity, its own personality, and a lot of fun. I love going over there.

Corey: I've seen documentaries on brothels in Nevada from the 70s and I look at the women working here now. What made the transition? Because the women back then looked like the kind of women you'd find hanging out at the laundromat.

Hof: Nevada has always been known for that: sex is available and the girls are really pretty sad. They're there because they can't do anything else. We've changed that drastically. Most of Nevada is still like that. At the Love Ranch and the BunnyRanch, it's not like that. What changed it? We opened the doors to the media so people could see. Remember when people are watching our TV show and the wife saying, "It's not so bad. Wow. I kind of like that place" so are their daughters. They're watching us and thinking, "That ain't so bad. I can do that. I want to have fun." Nearly every email I get, "I want to have fun with team BunnyRanch." Mom and dad's watch and are like, "That isn't so bad" and the daughters are like, "I'm gonna be a Bunny." That changed it big time. Opening the doors to the media and allowing them to see what's really going on here. Everybody's been here. Diane Sawyer's been here. *The Today Show. New Yorker* magazine did eleven pages. Everybody's been here and done something and it's always a different twist so we keep it interesting. The second thing is opening the Ranch up to porn girls. Porn girls would just quietly do things on the side. It would never be public about what they were doing. The producers and the companies, especially the bigger ones like Vivid, Wicked and VCA didn't want any part of that. "No. You're gonna be a hooker? We don't want any part of you." So, the girls had to do it quietly. They couldn't publicize it. Some of them did. Some of them didn't. When Sunset Thomas came here, I took this nationwide. I did press releases, took her on Howard Stern at the time. Howard had like 18 million people, that opened it all up. She came in here, worked here for six days and booked nearly a hundred thousand dollars. She got some heat in Los Angeles and it's like, "Excuse me? You girls are here blowing guys on camera for 600 bucks - a thousand bucks. I went up there and did less sex than I do on a set for a four-day movie and I made 45...50 thousand dollars. You think whatever the hell you want to think." So, all of a sudden, the girls are like, "Wow. Can that really be done?" Yes. We could do it legally so more and more came...Teri

Weigel came and just lots and lots of names. The more girls that came, the better it got in and opened up. It's okay. Finally, the guys like Larry Flynt, who is my friend, said, "What's the problem here?" He came out and said, "What's the problem? The girls are doing this stuff on the side. Why shouldn't they go do it legally with the proper protection and licensing and they're paying taxes." He said, "You guys got it wrong here and that's it." Seven hundred girls have been here.

Corey: Are there people you asked to come work or hinted to them that they should come work and they've hemmed and hawed?

Hof: When you're the hottest chick in the disco, you don't ask people to go home with you. They ask you. I'm the hottest chick in the disco with the BunnyRanch. Now did I ask a couple girls? Yes. I did ask a couple girls and I didn't get a response. I assume the answer's no. What I said was, "Lindsay Lohan and Britney (Spears) and Paris Hilton, you're out there giving this stuff away. You are giving away twenty million dollars' worth. Come sell it. Wise up. You can give the money to charity." If Britney would have been here selling it; she wouldn't have hooked up with the idiot Kevin and she would be where she is today. She would have been hotter. She can't compete with these girls. She's gotta get her body right. She'd have to look good and stay on top of her game to compete. Those are the only three girls I've ever really actively solicited and asked people to reach out to them. Wise up girls. Wake up. Don't give this away anymore. Come on. Come to the BunnyRanch. Have fun.

Corey: I didn't realize that Isabella Soprano had done some porn work before she came here.

Hof: No.

Corey: That was after?

Hof: Yes. She came here and she hooked up with Rayveness. She wanted to do some porn and I said, "No. Don't do it. Your career is just blowing up now. Let's make the money. If you're going to do it; I'll take you and we'll do it right." Because what they really want is the notoriety. They want to be a star porn star. Every chick that's ever had a camera on her and masturbated is a porn star. If I started saying Bunny Star, more people would want to be it. Three thousand girls a month apply. I'm gonna make you a Bunny Star. There's something about that word star which is actually bullshit. In the porn business you can count the stars on one hand. It's really simple. There are only a few stars then there's the girls that have done some movies. She wanted to do that. She went down, got in porn world and she did skank porn. This difference between classy porn and features and skank. She did skank porn. I didn't like it. I told her so. Then she got a drug habit and she couldn't kick it. She rehabbed. It didn't work. We kept bringing her up to be in the show, but we didn't want her working like that. She got out of that business and she's picking organic vegetables in Massachusetts. She's got no money and I heard she's pregnant. This is a girl that could have made a million dollars in a year. She could have been the highest-paid bunny ever. Air Force Amy makes a half a million dollars every year. She could have made a real million dollars in one year. Because she went down and got in the porn industry and got involved with the wrong people. There's good and bad to every business...it happened that she got involved with some bad people and ruined her career. She was the most popular person on our show. More than Sunset, even more than Air Force Amy. You know every day of my life; I get asked about Air Force Amy. It used to be Isabella. I get asked about her even more. We get maybe five to eight hundred requests for her a month right now. She's not here. (*Editor's Note: The interview has been on Youtube for over a decade and Isabella Soprano has never contacted me to give her side of the story.*)

Corey: I look at Katie Morgan and what she's been able to do off the *Pornucopia* series. I get a sense that HBO would have given Isabella the same treatment.

Hof: Yes, if she had been...yes, absolutely, absolutely. Katie's done a great job.

Brooke Taylor
Interview

Brooke: But you want me to talk directly in the camera?

Corey: Yes. Talk directly. This is for the internet.

Brooke: I just didn't know if you wanted my eyeline to be it.

Corey: We should talk about how you become very professional and very more understanding of eyelines. In a way you're a TV personality, but you still have your day job? How is the balance of that?

Brooke: It's an interesting balance. You learn as you go along. Just like I learned here in the bedroom as I went along, I learned a little bit from every television show or any interview I do. I just try to be a good Hooker and take it all with me.

Corey: When people come to visit, are they taken back that the HBO cameras aren't here?

Brooke: A lot of people think that the HBO cameras would be here. We have to explain they're only here at certain times and you have to sign a waiver. We can't just put you on TV. You got to be aware of it. There's so many people begging me in emails all the time, "Can I be one of your regulars so I can do a scene with you?" We're getting the word out there that we're not invaded by cameras.

Corey: I saw a warning sign pointing out that the HBO cameras aren't here.

Brooke: Yeah, yeah. People want to be discreet and we want to keep it discreet so we let them know that they're not here.

Corey: In the first episode, you came here, had your first party and then you called your mom.

Brooke: I called my mom.

Corey: How has the relationship with your mom progressed as your notoriety has progressed?

Brooke: My relationship with my mom is wonderful and always has been. She is my biggest fan and a wonderful support system for me. My father now knows. At the time I made that phone call to my mother; my father didn't know. Now he does and he's supportive as well. This season you'll see my mom actually come out and take her first visit to the

BunnyRanch. She doesn't work though. I wouldn't let her.

Corey: So, no mother-daughter tandems?

Brooke: No mother-daughter tandems. My mom is not a MILF. I mean, God bless her and I love her. But she's not a MILF. I'm sorry.

Corey: You're on the cover of *Hustler* and inside *Marie Claire* at the same time. Talk to me about going between high-fashion and *Hustler*.

Brooke: I didn't just make the cover of Hustler. I'm the cover and centerfold which is pretty much unheard. That was such an honor. Sometimes it's difficult when you're in prostitution to finally feel accepted in the adult industry as far as the magazines. I haven't done pornography, but um I guess everything I do is pornography. I haven't done any videos. It's hard to feel as accepted and that sort of secured myself in the sex industry as being acknowledged for providing a great service. Then the exact opposite to go to Marie Claire which focuses less on my physical appearance and more on me, my background and what brought me here. In the same month I got extremes and you get to see all sides of me. It was great and I like it.

Corey: Which magazine did you send mom first?

Brooke: Mom actually got sent the Hustler first because that's the one I received first. I had an advance copy of that so mom definitely got the

Hustler first. Kind of like my birth, she saw me nude before I could talk. So, it's sort of the same way.

Corey: *The Morning Show with Mike and Juliet* (a Fox syndicated TV show) wants you back as a regular guest.

Brooke: *The Mike and Juliet* show is a wonderful show to do. I think they were a little surprised by how... I don't want to toot my own horn...but how educated I am. I can put together a complete sentence. I can defend myself and change people's opinions about this business. They've invited me to come back on and I'm very excited. (*Editor's note: The Morning Show with Mike and Juliet was canceled in June of 2009. Juliet Huddy would settle a sexual harassment lawsuit against Fox News that involved Bill O'Reilly and Fox News co-president Jack Abernethy.*)

Corey: You and Dennis are a unique tandem. People are used to guys who run a house like this and the people who work there to not being defensible and more being caricatures. Do you think you've ushered in a new level of how people approach the business?

Brooke: I think over the years America has been shocked by different sexual fetishes. Sex is so in-your-face now that it doesn't shock them anymore. Where it's benefited me is showing people that I don't fit into the stereotypes of a typical prostitute and Dennis doesn't fit into those stereotypes of a pimp. That's served me very well and it does change people's opinion about this business which it should. This business can be a great asset to the community. They're not aware of how it works and the people who work there. The process of it all. They'll never know and if it comes time for them to vote; they now at least have all the information now.

Corey: How's your time at the house changed with your higher profile? Do you do more pre-arranged dates?

Brooke: I've been very lucky in providing a good service from day one. I have a good base of clients that take care of me and I take care of them. Most of the time if you were to walk in the doors, I might be milling around here and you can ask for me. But I don't always run to the line. Don't tell anyone. So, the best way is to make an appointment with me and that way I always make sure I'm available for you. Plus, you get more bang for your buck by taking your time out to specifically come and see me. I've been very lucky that way for a couple of years.

Corey: How much time do you spend on the road doing promotions?

Brooke: My time on the road really depends on the month. Depends on what's going on. I'll be on the road more if a story like the Governor Spitzer thing comes out again or if we have a new television show coming out. It just really depends. Month by month, it's different and that's really what I like about this job because no two days are ever the same and no two months are ever alike.

Corey: I'm guessing you didn't expect any of this when you initially wrote to Dennis and said, "Hey, I want to work here."

Brooke: No. I just expected to make enough money to go to grad school. I've made that sum. But ya know I never imagined that my life would take the turns that it has. But I firmly believe that life will take you where you need to go whether you think you need to go there or not. I'm just enjoying being her.

Corey: I've heard you have been performing after *Cathouse The Musical* special.

Brooke: I have been performing. *Cathouse The Musical* really broke me out of my shy shell of singing. I've been exploiting that talent as best as I can. I really love performing and I love being on stage. I do have a degree in music. So, music has always been very near and dear to me and a big part of my life. It's really exciting to see how coming to the BunnyRanch, something really seemingly far off for music, can ultimately tie me back in and propel me to the next level. I'm really excited.

Corey: Where have you been performing live?

Brooke: I have been performing live. I performed at the House of Blues in Hollywood twice, the Hard Rock in Las Vegas and the Fillmore in San Francisco. I'm gonna be going in the studio and working with a wonderful producer, Mark Hudson (of the Hudson Brothers) this month. I'm really excited. I'll get to display all my oral skills. The things that come out, not just go in.

Corey: When I interviewed you the first time, I joked about the idea of getting a hold of the episode and cutting just the musical moments so you can show them to relatives without having to be squeamish. Did you ever do a G-Rated cut?

Brooke: I never did a G-Rated cut. I've given up on protecting the family. If they want to see, they can see it. They can close our eyes. They're smart enough to figure out when something's coming up. I'm just living my life andI have been very blessed that my family is so accepting and loving. It really is unconditional support that I have from them. They get the full version. They can edit it themselves. I don't have time.

Corey: What keeps you stable? You're recording music, you're on TV and you have your day job here. What keeps you stable from not falling completely into some sort of unreality bliss?

Brooke: Mom and dad keep me stable. I mean especially mom. I mean we talk so many times. I've already talked to her twice today. She really is my best friend and you can't float away when it comes to your mom. She's always gonna keep you in check. She's always gonna let you know how it is and tell it like it is. She always has your best interest at heart even if it's not what you want to hear. It's definitely my family. Just knowing where I come from keeps me grounded.

Corey: What would you recommend to any woman who watches the show and wants to write into Denis and say, "Hey, this is the life for me!" What would you tell them are the good parts and things you don't see on camera that you need to be prepared for?

Brooke: If this is something you want to do, you just need to make sure that it is something you want to do. Know your boundaries before coming. Know whether or not you want to do media or you want to keep it discreet. And stick to them. Nobody can make the decision except for you. Nobody knows that this is the right thing for you to do except for yourself. Follow your gut. Follow your heart. If this is where you're supposed to be, I'm sure you'll have a great time while you're at it.

Corey: I noticed while here that there's a lot of waiting.

Brooke: Oh yeah. There is a lot of waiting. That's probably one thing in the job that people don't realize. You read a lot of books and play a lot of board games. You need to keep yourself occupied and motivated while you're here. Negotiation is not as easy as you would think it is. So, study study study. Read your book. Practice. It's very easy to slip into a lackadaisical way of living around here. You always want to make sure that you remain focused with your goals in mind. And set goals. A lot of girls don't set goals and don't let it just be those new Gucci shoes. Have a purpose in life and get yourself there.

Corey: What are your goals?

Brooke: My goals...I have so many goals. My goal is to be successful at music and be happy in life. Just enjoy every last day. It kind of seems like I don't have goals, but those in themselves are goals because as far as career and where I'm going that way, the options are endless. I can't limit myself and I would be here all day if I listed my career goal.

Corey: You've done a lot. You have a degree in music. You come here away from the Square World and you're achieving those goals. You're performing at the Filmore and the House of Blues. How easy is it for you to look around and think, "This is too weird but I'm enjoying it?"

Brooke: I think it sinks in little by little what I'm doing and I don't think all of it has quite sunk in yet. You really do just have to take it all in and enjoy every last moment. Sometimes I feel like being pinched. I'll even tell people, Pinch me. I feel like

I'm dreaming." But it's wonderful that we live in a world where when you really put your mind to doing something, you can live in that dream state and be that happy. I'm one of the few people in this world that actually enjoys their job. Truly a hundred percent so I'm very lucky for that.

Corey: Do you also find it strange because *Cathouse* is one of the few reality TV shows that the home viewer can wander into without worrying about beating up on the security guard. A guy sitting at home can go, "Oh, I'd like to be with her." He can make a phone call--

Brooke: And come be with me.

Corey: Yeah. You've been to those reality award shows and you know there's no way any of those people are going to take the phone call and say, "Come out and pal around with me."

Brooke: I have noticed a difference in my clientele. It's not very often when someone comes in and it hasn't seen me on something. It's interesting because sometimes it's hard for someone who watches me on TV to understand that I'm not watching them back. Sometimes I worry if I am living up to their expectations of who I am or their idea of who they thought I was. I just do my best to be myself and that's what I do when the cameras are here. That's what I do when the cameras aren't here. So far, it's worked well. I think it's really neat that I can share myself with people in a different way that actresses, other musicians, and people in society can't. I find it to be an honor and a privilege. I'll keep screwing my customers cuz they seem to enjoy it as much as I do.

Corey: In a weird way you're not a sex symbol because there's nothing symbolic about what you do. You're not unattainable to those who see and enjoy you.

Brooke: I am attainable. There still are people out there who maybe don't know our pricing. They think because I'm on TV, I might be too expensive. I think that having that allure of the unattainable is kind of what men like. Here's the one place that the woman they never thought in a million years they could ever have is. Here I am just waiting for you. I'm just sitting on my bed playing with a puppy, waiting for you to come in.

Corey: Does it also help you in a weird way because they have this image of you as a TV star and so when you turn your attention on them, they melt?

Brooke: Men always melted for me. To me it doesn't matter whether you've seen me on TV or not. I'm gonna be the same person with you regardless. But it is very flattering, and it does boost my self-esteem when someone gets really giddy around you. Knowing that you can make someone feel like that little school kid again on the playground, it's a good feeling. It's fun.

Corey: I know I've asked about the Tiffany episode before, but do people ask you, "Was that woman for real?" (editor's note: Tiffany was a woman who showed up at the BunnyRanch and refused to perform oral sex on clients).

Brooke: People ask me about Tiffany. T they asked me if we're sisters and I'm like, "Yeah. She's the garbage from my mom cuz I give blowjobs and she doesn't. The funny thing about that episode, I was brand new. I had no idea. When I saw the episode, I thought, "Is this for real?" But yes, she was for real. Dennis seems to think she was here to put the move on him and maybe she was. I think she was just trying to see what she could get away with. Exploiting HBO and Cathouse for what it is. But regardless of whether that's the real her or not; it was very entertaining. I hope I never see her again. I'll just have a dick in my mouth every time or I'm just gonna grab a dildo and suck on it every time I'm around her.

Corey: Are you surprised you haven't seen her on *The Flavor of Love*?

Brooke: Maybe I did see her on *The Flavor of Love*. Every now and again I browse Craigslist. I'm just waiting. She'll come out with porn or something. I don't know what her deal was. She left in the middle of the night and never made a dime. For as wonderful as she was; nobody got to find out.

Corey: Do other reality TV shows approach you to come on as a guest star or a *Surreal Life* kind of situation?

Brooke: I haven't been approached to do *The Surreal Life* or other reality television shows yet. So far, it's just been news shows and talk shows and things of that nature. Hey I'm up for it. If someone needs a cameo hooker role in some movie or something somewhere along the lines. Maybe I'll even get killed off. That would be cool. So, you never know. (Editor's Note: It doesn't appear Brooke was ever a hooker on *CSI*. But she did end up on an episode of *Oprah* in 2009.)

Corey: Well, thank you so much.

Brooke: Thank you.

November 16th, 2010

Call it Hof Vegas. Dennis Hof of HBO's *Cathouse* no longer wants me to warn readers that his BunnyRanch empire is in only Reno and not Las Vegas. He's bringing his style of adult fun to the outskirts of Sin City. He called up the hotline from the middle of Crystal, Nevada to spread the news. The sounds of hammering and drills came from his end of the phone.

"We're moving around here and getting some things done," Dennis Hof said. "I bought two 35-year-old rundown, rat trap brothels. What you're buying is the licenses."

The two old names were Cherry Patch Ranch and Mabel's Whore House. The new places are Love Ranch and Dennis Hof's Cathouse. "Those are names that are *synonymous* with good times."

There are no good times for the former owner. He got arrested for bribing a county official. Dennis found himself in a unique position to double up his business.

"He had to sell the place," Dennis said. "There's not a worse time in American history to sell a brothel. Nobody has any money. Nobody is investing in any businesses. I came in and bought the two places. I'm going through a massive renovation. I'm going to make it all work. Do my magic. I'm doing the same thing I did to the Bunny Ranch 18 years ago except I'm doing in Southern Nevada where the weather is better in the winter."

This is extremely true since it can be in the mid-80s in Las Vegas while Reno freezes. The new location also means exposure to more tourists than the number that visit the Biggest Little City in the World.

"The difference is instead of having 8 million people to draw from in Reno-Tahoe, I've got 40 million in Las Vegas," Hof said. He's realistic in his projection about how many people will want to visit his new houses. "We don't need that much. If you got 10 percent of 40 million, you got 4 million clients. I can't handle that. If you got one percent, it's 400,000. I can't handle that. If you get a tenth of one percent, that's 40,000 clients a year. That's fine. That's what I need."

For a few years there was sense that legal brothels would be allowed inside the city limits of Las Vegas. In the end the politicians couldn't allow this vice to taint their Sin City. Hof's two new brothels are the closest legal locations to the Strip. There's plenty of illegal action in the casinos and hotels. The city is filled with ads for ladies promising In Room Entertainment. They're not magicians, but they will perform plenty of tricks. Of course, the strangest trick is a transformation as they rarely appear as the performer promised. Is Las Vegas ready for a business where the woman on the website looks like the one you have the date with?

"I'm going to make them ready for me," Hof declared. "My new campaign is Las Vegas: America's Sexual Cesspool. What happens in Las Vegas, you take home to your wife. I've got lots of ammo to back that up. In Nevada, the legal business in 30 years of mandatory checks has never had a case of HIV. The illegal business in Las Vegas, there's been 400 girls arrested and forced to take a test and shown to have HIV. It's horrifying. I'm going to change all that.

"The city needs to be outed for enabling all this to happen. The mayor comes out and says there's 3,000 active pimps working in Las Vegas and 30,000 girls. If you know that, do something about it. And if you don't do something about it and your tourists are getting diseases, aren't you responsible for it?"

Hof wants people who contract VD in Las Vegas to sue the city for refusing to allow the legal brothel system to operate in city limits while the illegal prostitution rackets thrive. "It's a far-out concept. But I don't know if it is or not."

He's quite happy in his new location of the small town of Crystal. It's not too far away from Vegas. "Depends on how you come and where you're at," Hof said. "If you're close to Freemont, it's 45 minutes. If you're in the heart of Las Vegas and coming through Pahrump, it's an hour."

The population of Crystal is only 107 but expect that number to grow.

"We got a dozen girls now. Eight working and four on vacation. When we get more rooms done, we'll expand to the next level," Hof said. It's very hard to create an intimate mood with a "Pardon Our Dust" sign above the bed.

"We want the place to look nice and the girls to be proud of where they're working. We're working hard on it. It's going to be great. I don't have the same construction constraints that I have up there. Here I can plan this paradise as a beautiful resort destination with a swimming pool, Jacuzzis and palm trees."

You should be able to watch the progress of Dennis Hof's *Cathouse* thanks to his new neighbor: Heidi Fleiss. She's helping him on the reality show about upgrading the old buildings. *Extreme Ho House Makeover* is the current title. Although I suggested the more direct *Pimp My Brothel.*

There were reports on the internet that Hof was marrying Heidi Fleiss. Hof explained how the rumored nuptials happened. "That goes back a few years ago when Heidi got out of *Celebrity Rehab.* She flashbacked on when we split up." She thought Dennis was going to marry her, but he said he couldn't marry someone on drugs. He told her that when she's off drugs, they'd talk about it. "She had this flashback and put out a press release saying that we were getting married. And I'm like 'What the fuck are you doing?' She said, 'You told me.' I said, 'You're right. I absolutely did say that. But I'm not in the marrying mood right now.'"

This explains why you didn't hear about them being registered at Crate and Barrel.

Hof is still a relatively single man although he's hooked up with Cami Parker.

"Cami is wonderful," Hof said. "She likes girls so we get along really well with that. Girlfriend in my vernacular is the girl I sleep with the most. I tend to wake up with her more than anybody."

She's also his second girlfriend in a row that's found herself featured in *Hustler*. How did this honor come about?

"Went to lunch with her and Larry Flint and he fell in love with her," Hof admits.

Air Force Amy, Brooke Taylor and Dennis ended up on episodes of *Judge Jeanine Pirro*. Dennis was collecting from a deadbeat client that didn't think he had to pay for a girl-girl show. It was interesting to note that under normal legal circumstances, Dennis would be the defendant. But here he was using the law to get what's owed.

"Ain't that something," Hof said. "What a turn around that is. I've taken this business from guilt and shame to glamour and fame. If you're a Bunny Ranch girl now, you're walking through an airport, they love you. Eighteen years ago, nobody would admit you worked at the Bunny Ranch."

Cathouse favorite Air Force Amy isn't hanging around any of the houses at the current time. "She's gone. We have a love-hate relationship with Amy. We love her when she's clean and sober. When the twelve-step program doesn't work, the thirteenth step is out the door. If she straightens out, we got something to talk about."

Those interested in meeting adult superstar Sunny Lane need to make an appointment. "Sunny hasn't been working much. She's been doing a few more movies and fell in love. This year she's backed off some."

The legendary Chasey Lane has signed up to work in Crystal, but there's a hitch.

"She has not got here yet," Hof said. "We're taking appointments for her. We're trying to find out what her arrest record is. She doesn't even know. She went through a little wild child stage. We're trying to get that all worked out. Each county in Nevada has different rules. The county by Las Vegas, if you have a marijuana arrest, it's OK long as you haven't gotten in trouble since then. Our county in Northern Nevada says no. We want you to wait five years. That's the way it is. She is going to work. It's just which place and how soon."

Southwest Air flies to both Vegas and Reno so you can change your flight depending where she ends up.

"Whomever parties with this girl will not forget it," Hof promised. You'll be humming "The Ballad of Chasey Lain" by the Bloodhound Gang afterward.

Joe Pesci and Helen Mirren's *Love Ranch* caused a bit of controversy when the producers attempted to go after Dennis for naming his second brothel the Love Ranch. Dennis wasn't backing down since the screenwriter got the name from Dennis. Turns out that things worked themselves out without a protracted legal battle. Also didn't hurt that the film completely tanked over the summer.

"It's a shame they didn't make some money cause I would have got a bunch of it," Hof said. "It is my federal trademark, but I cut them some slack. Taylor Hackford (the director) acknowledged me at the premiere and had me stand up. That was nice of him."

Dennis plans on stocking DVDs of *Love Ranch* in the gift shops of his two Love Ranches. He'll probably end up making more money than the producers.

Also, on the shelves of the gift shops are bottles of Dennis' award-winning hot sauce. They are as hot on the label as the contents. "The Bunny of the month gets her own hot sauce. They're turning into collector's items. The girls sign them," Hof said. With any luck, he'll be starting a hot sauce of the month club for folks who want heat on their spice rack. You can get more info on the sauce by visiting Loveranch.net and bunnyranch.com.

In a time where companies are refusing to grow that Hof is doubling his business. Although by giving clients a Love Ranch in both cities, he can save money by doubling up orders of matchbooks and business cards. He's also figuring out ways to be in two places on the same day.

"I'm going back and forth as needed. What I need to do is buy an airplane. I'm going to charter a plane for a while to see if I really enjoy it as much as I think

I will." The road between Reno and Vegas takes him about 6 hours versus a barely two-hour trip by air.

Strangely enough there is no nickname for people who live between Reno and Vegas. Bi-Vadian is my suggestion.

Hof boosted the local economy when he purchased numerous mattresses for the new locations at the locally owned Building 160.

"We want to spend money where we make it. We want to buy things in that community. We want to give back to the community. It's been a successful formula for 18 years. I love it that way."

The recent bedbug infestation news can have nasty consequences in an industry that relies heavily on mattresses. "One of the reasons we got rid of them all is we're scared to death of bedbugs. One of the mattresses we threw away had a sticker from 1978 on it. How much action has that mattress seen? Most of these mattresses were worn out ten years ago."

There are no plans yet for Hof to make a guest appearance on *Pawn Stars*. "I should do that," Hof declared. "Bring some brothel memorabilia over there." It will be TV history with the meeting of Bunny Love with Chumlee. With any luck, they'd become a reality TV could nicknamed ChumLove.

The next installment of HBO's *Cathouse* is slated for December 16. "Our ninth year. Can you believe it?" Dennis points out. "And we're going to do a tenth year." The show is still one of the highest viewed options on HBO's OnDemand channel. *Cathouse: The Specials* comes out on DVD the Tuesday before the new episode.

In the midst of the job crisis, Dennis is getting plenty of resumes from around the country. What helps an applicant get to the top of the pile? "Personality, People skills, desire, hotness…. the hotness is all subjective. People skills, personality and desire rules."

There are also traits that get instant rejection. "People who have substance abuse issues. Drama. If they can't live in a dormitory-type environment," Hof listed.

Age is not an issue. "As long as a girl takes care of herself," Hof qualified. "Some people look pretty hot at different ages."

While the southern version of the Love Ranch is operating, it will be a little bit longer before the grand opening of Dennis Hof's Cathouse. "Probably six months," he projected. "I'm working with the architect right now. When we go, we're going big and fast with the construction."

Will there be a Subway subs next to the new gift shop? Dennis had joked in the past that he bought the Bunny Ranch because Subway wouldn't let him acquire a franchise. Will Jared be cutting the ribbon to open up the Cathouse?

"After all these years, Subway should be begging me to have one," Dennis said. "I'm going to open up a restaurant there. It's going to basically be a Waffle House. I love Waffle House. I think every guy does. It's quick, clean, convenient, filling and the price is right. I'm going to open up a mini-Waffle House. Same kind of menu."

Speaking from experience, Sunday morning waffles with the bunnies ought to be on your bucket list. It is so much better than breakfast with the Disney characters. Just be careful with what you do with the syrup.

Besides his own show and construction, Dennis is helping two productions about the horrors of prostitution in Las Vegas. The city is notorious for underaged girls and smuggled in illegal aliens from Eastern Europe.

"Once they understand the risks for disease, that's enough to get you to drive 45 minutes," Hof said. "When you call a girl in Las Vegas, you don't know if you're going to get a cop."

We joke about him hiring any ex-female cops for clients that have a fetish about being caught in a sting.

Ultimately Dennis Hof wants to fill the void left by the death of Danny Gans. He's aiming to be the number one entertainer. He wants to put the Sin back in Sin City without the annoying rash.

October 30th, 2012

Dennis Hof is transforming. He has a bordello empire with a license to operate a sixth house in the works. He'll have more women working for his houses than players in the NBA. He just opened the Alien Cathouse near Area 51. This new themed establishment makes it possible for nerds to truly hook up with a woman in a Princess Leia Slave Ensemble. He has a new knee and girlfriend (naturally a blonde) helping him rehab. He's ready to party and his birthday's the perfect excuse to celebrate.

How could the Party Favors refuse an invitation to spend a weekend celebration in the World Famous Bunny Ranch within craps throwing distance of

Reno? The good part about a Dennis Hof party is that it's not going to end up a sausage fest. There shall be ladies and interesting guests. This is what your friends in college imagined their parties were going to be like…except they weren't like a Dennis Hof party. I couldn't miss out on the fun since I needed to perform more research for my upcoming business book: *House Rules: How to Make Your Employees Love Being Treated As Prostitutes*. The self-help book is based on my experiences with Dennis over the years. Forget Donald Trump as a business role model. Dennis has mastered the concept of making everybody happy at the end of a deal.

The party was set up to be a three day blow out. Madame Suzette had planned out a celebration worthy of her boss's stature as the place to party. This wasn't only going to be cake, ice cream, punch and a few party favors. There will be things that won't be allowed on Instagram. Down in the Southern part of Nevada, they have an old tourism board saying, "What Happens in Vegas, Stays in Vegas." But what's the deal with Carson City? How much can I tell about a "lost weekend" in a brothel? The Party Favors decided that if Dennis mentioned it as part of his Ustream show, it's fair game to relate. I'm not going to tease you that much - this isn't about going to a stripclub. This was the greatest party since Truman Capote's Black and White Ball.

Friday night was the social evening of drinks and karaoke to let the guests. `There was a great delight in just hanging out in the lobby and bar chatting away while Dennis welcomed his friends to his dream house. Dennis moved very well for a man who had knee replacement surgery six weeks before. But he also has the greatest rehab partners to keep him interested in therapy. His latest girlfriend is Courtney Cross, a tall Texas blond with a surprising talent. More on that later. What happened to his last girlfriend that was featured on HBO's *Cathouse*? No need to ask. All you need to know is that Dennis Hof is the only man in America who doesn't whine about getting back in the dating scene. He has better things to discuss in conversations. He mentioned how he explained to Elizabeth Taylor the difference between a vibrator and a dildo. My ears quickly perk up with such a tale. Dennis did once dine with the first lady of cinema. Ron Jeremy wanted to sleep with her so he could brag about the occasion. Naturally he wouldn't point out what year it happened. A lot of the talk focused on Andy Kaufman. The late star of *Taxi* was Dennis' traveling partner to Nevada cathouses in the late '70s. How come that wasn't in *The Man In the Moon*? I swore Tony Clifton's ghost roamed around the hot tub in the back during the weekend. Or maybe it really was Tony Clifton.

The big talk of this visit to Ranch was "The Girlfriend Experience." Not sure what influence the movie played in the craze, but seems like a lot of men I met had their prime lady to see. There are a few women working exclusively as the girlfriend experience. They only visit the ranch when their date flies into town for a weekend long date. They don't come running when the bell rings for the line-up. One guy explained to me that the girlfriend experience is cheaper by the hour than his last divorce lawyer. He kept in contact with his "girlfriend" over the internet between his flights to the Reno-Tahoe airport. The only bad difficult part of "the experience" is a chance of relationship drama. Some girlfriends don't like seeing their "boyfriends" disappearing into other rooms. But when you're a kid in a candy store, you can't resist sampling from other colorful jars.

I quickly found myself enjoying the "Friend Who's a Girl Experience" with the stunning Bailey Paige. The tall blond had remembered me from four years earlier when interviewed Dennis for the award winning "Hof/Corey Interview." We quickly became drinking buddies for what turned out to be a longer night than I expected with a body still on east coast time. Casinos pump pure oxygen through the air vents to keep gamblers throwing around the chips. I have my suspicion that Dennis has figured out how to turn Red Bull into an aerosol spray to keep the party bouncing until the wee hours.

During the first night festivities, Dennis introduced me to Sunny Lane. How can I talk about Sunny without sounding so sunny? How do you even talk to her? The AVN winning actress is a rarity amongst adult performers with her lack of surgical enhancements. She has a body made for HDTV. The

Georgia Peach grew up with dreams of being an Olympic ice skater. That dream fell through when issues with her feet that took her off the ice. Through a series of circumstances, she landed a job at the Bunny Ranch and appeared on the early episodes of *Cathouse* as Sunshine. This led to a career in adult cinema including the new *Batgirl XXX*. Here's the almost workplace safe version of the trailer.

I became locked into awkward teenage mindset of muttering, "You're so purty." This however did not destroy the encounter. Sunny guided me on a tour of all the changes Dennis made since the last visit. There's a brand-new heated pool that's perfect for late night skinny dips. The hot tub has been upgraded. The bunnies are happy to have a larger work out center. There's even a corral for Dennis' horses. During the day, wild horses visit the compound. It's truly the nature scene on the hill. It was a chilly night and Sunny was dressed in her skimpy work outfit. I loaned her my sweatshirt. We marveled at how bright the stars were in the Nevada sky. As I looked back down and saw her bundled inside my sweatshirt, I pondered if this moment was the "Gosh I Should Ask You Out to See If You'd Like to be My Girlfriend Experience." She is such a sweetheart. She had taken a break from movies and working at the Bunny Ranch to enjoy life, but is now back and full of steam. Even with such an adorable cuteness, there's a focused drive to her eyes. She is serious about her career in the flesh trade. She spoke of the issues in the adult video industry including the various sites offering free streams of her life's work. This was what drove her to wake up in the wee small hours of the night to check the sharpness of her blades.

Sunny spoke about her time meeting Kim Kardashian. She'd figure they'd bond since they both are known for their asses and sex tapes. But Kim wanted nothing to do with Sunny. This is probably just pure envy on Kim's part since Sunny knows how to work her ass and looks like she's enjoys getting laid in her sex tapes. Sunny should have her own E! series since her mom and dad help with her career. Why can't Ryan Secrest give us "Sunny Side Up!" or something of that ilk-ish titling?

During our tour, we stopped by the room of Caressa Kisses. A lot of people ask what kind of woman works at the Bunny Ranch. Mostly they expect tales of high school drop outs that went to work at Hooters, moved up to strip clubs and adult movies until they ended up in prostitution. Carrasa surprised me when she spoke of working in an operating room. I foolishly asked if she was a surgical nurse. She's a surgeon. Why is she operating for Dennis? She went through med school and finished her residency. Her student debt was enormous. Instead of living on Top Ramen while paying off massive loans and huge malpractice insurance premiums, Carrasa called up Madame Suzette. She is a doctor who has bedroom eyes.

During the three-way conversation, Sunny mentioned how much she likes Carrasa and it'd be really cool if we had a threesome.

Leonard Cohen should have written "The Sisters of Mercy" about these two ladies. There was such a warmth and spiritual healing feeling between them. As they both smiled at me, I could sense that this would be the kind of event that I'd brag about on my deathbed to loved ones before they smothered me with a pillow. It wasn't just going to be a dirty evening, but a religious experience. A surgeon's hands and a flexible figure skater made me think that this would be a party that had to last all weekend. Could I afford the Caligula dream that was kicking against my frontal lobes? Why didn't I start a hedge fund? How much would they give me for my spare kidney? What if I threw in a spleen? Does my family need to eat for the rest of the year? Didn't we eat enough food in the summer? Where are my magic beans? Will my wife bury me in a shallow grave or dump me in the lake "Dexter"-style? The sad truth is that the Party Favors expense account no longer covers Hookers and Blow like in the '80s. My accountant warned me that even if I reviewed the party in the Party Favors, the IRS would cut me up if I claimed it as a business expense. For a brief moment, I prayed that Patti Kaplan would scratch on the door to let me know HBO was picking up the tab if I agreed to let them film it. But there was no Make A Wish miracle. Nobody at Mastercard had to wonder if I put a down payment on buying Costa Rica. I was there to report and not play Neil Strauss. This is the most painful "fish that got away" story since I busted open my knee diving to catch an escaping bass. But at least I'm telling it to you and not a bankruptcy judge wondering how I spent two weeks in a bed. He'd probably want illustrations and I'd give them. Give me a minute to stop crying. What's wrong with sending the kid to Community College and living in a tent? It builds character. Sunny guided me out of Carassa's room. It was a walk of shame for me. But at least Sunny was wearing my sweatshirt.

Back at the bar, the karaoke was in full swing. I found out more about the background of various Bunnies. One, whose name will remain secret, was on fall break from grad school. Her two weeks at the Ranch were going to cover spring semester. Tegan Tate was a trip since she reminded me of the Dark Side of *Juno*. The pixie-ish porn star had recently arrived at the Ranch after making a few films for the saintly folks at San Francisco's Kink.com. What do you say to a woman that has "Punish me" tattooed under her breast? Sadie Lee talked to me about how she tried for a few weeks being a mail-order prostitute. She'd get appointments and fly around the country. She didn't like the fact that she didn't know who lurked behind the hotel room door and what he really wanted for his money. She liked the safety of Dennis' bordello.

Hard to tell why HBO hasn't done a new special about the Bunny Ranch. There are so many stories eager to spill out from behind the gate. Patti Kaplan could make an entire special about Jayla Conrad, a third-generation ranch hand. The redhead told me how when she was 16, she came across material from the Moonlite Ranch featuring not only her mom, but her grandmother. She waited until after Thanksgiving dinner to ask her mom and grandma. They didn't deny it. We wondered if there's ever a good time to let a daughter know that you and grandma worked at a cathouse? Maybe the topic could be mentioned after an episode of *Cathouse*? Turns out mom didn't work there that long, but Jayda's aunt did. Dennis said that Jayda's aunt is responsible for getting him to buy the Moonlight Ranch and turning it into the Moonlite Bunny Ranch. Dennis also admitted to hooking up with Jayda's grandmother. Andy Kaufman was part of this family-style fun. How can HBO not see a "Cathouse: Family Tradition" special in Jayda's family story? They could run it next Thanksgiving. Get on it, Sheila Nivens!

Saturday night was the big party at Dennis' nightclub. The theme was alien costumes so the room was covered in lots of intergalactic naughtiness. Slutty alien described most of the wardrobe choices. The major shocker was that only one woman showed up in the Slave Leia outfit. For those wondering, I showed up in a white safe suit like the guys who investigate alien landings.

The big star of the night was none other than Ron Jeremy. Why hasn't the Kennedy Center Honored Ron Jeremy? The man has made more movies than Jimmy Stewart. He's even made a movie that doesn't feature him naked although those straight films have him being killed in various ways. It's pop or be popped in the cinema of Ron. He's not a tall guy. In fact, it felt odd towering over the living legend. Ron spent most of the night posing for pictures, signing breasts and eating at the buffet. The man enjoys his meals. Who couldn't resist the buffet since it featured Moon Pies! I was going to bring Dennis some of the tasty Southern treats, but feared the TSA would swipe them from my luggage.

Instead of just people merely hanging out, there was a floor show courtesy of some very talented Bunnies and gals from The Love Ranch. Acts included hula hoops, Brooke Taylor wearing a blond wig, Psy dancing and the Samba. The strangest moment was when Courtney Cross stepped on stage to deliver topless opera. People were expecting something on par with Bugs Bunny's "What's Opera, Doc?" Instead, Courtney delivered a moving aria with her serious operatic skills. She did lose her top to make sure the crowd paid proper attention. Another big pleasure was a photo booth set up. All night people struck triple posers that sometimes looked like a session for a Vivid Video cover. Here's a behind the angle of Sunny Lane (the blond) and Jayla Conrad (blue hair).

Singing in the background is Sadie Lee. She was my karaoke buddy from the previous night. Dennis' big birthday bash was all about bodies bumping into bodies without much complaining. There was body painting with no reservations as women completely stripped down to get the paint sprayed everywhere. Bailey only wanted a pair of wings painted on her back to give her more of angelic feel.

There were odd stars lurking at the party including "Arlo", an executive from *Hustler* and Andy Kaufman's pal Bob Zmuda. I'm standing with two people who have had their lives turned into supporting characters in Milos Foreman movies. They had been fictionalized into the faces of Crispin Glover and Paul Giamatti. I felt left out. Perhaps someday soon Milos will make a movie about Dennis Hof. Ryan Gosling will play me as the plucky internet columnist who brings his pregnant wife to the Bunny Ranch on their wedding anniversary. Although with my luck it'll be Kevin James. For the love of God, don't let Milos cast Tyler Perry as Medea as me. The after party back at the Bunny Ranch was even more exciting. You'd wonder when familiar faces disappeared if they'd gone to the bathroom or were enjoying an even more intimate after party. When you party in a bordello, anyone can get lucky at any time. This was better than being at the prom with a gallon of Jack Daniels and a canister of nitrous. The big fun came as I sat on the front porch with Mr. Dan Haggerty. He was the star of *The Life and Times of Grizzly Adams* which was a childhood favorite. He has a sideline marrying couples at the Bunny Ranch. He's tied the knot on over 200 parties with only one divorce. His big shocker of the night was telling us that he'd had a one-night stand with Phyllis Diller. That's right, Grizzly Adams hooked up with Fang's Wife. You want details?

He was on a talkshow with Barbi Benton (*Playboy After Dark*) and Phyllis Diller. Barbi had just broken up with Hugh Hefner. After the show, Haggerty joked that he'd love to hook up with Barbi, but he was heading home with Phyllis. The couple did head out. She mused, "Fang, if you could see me now." The comic star did have a major request for their romp. "Now you do me a favor Danny," she asked. "What's that?" Dan responded. "Let me lay on the bottom so the wrinkles around my eyes disappear behind my ears." She cared about Dan's image as well. "Don't you worry about a thing," she said. "I'll go out the fire escape not to ruin your career." "Are you kidding, this will be the best thing that ever happened to me," Dan declared. The moment has not faded from Dan's memory since each year an event brings it all back. "Every time I look at a Thanksgiving turkey on the table and those little white pompoms on the end of their legs, I remember Phyllis' feet sticking in the air with her little white socks. Oh my God, is this going to be with me forever?" He laughed.

The afterparty kept going with guests mingling with clients showing up to party with the on-duty Bunnies. The strange feeling is that at that moment guys in New York City and around Maine are living in panic that their names will be revealed by the Soccer Madame and Zumba Hooker. Yet there we were sitting on the front porch of a brightly lit brothel without a care about being frogwalked by the cops and branded by shameful *New York Post* headlines. Dennis Hof has created a sanctuary on the outskirts of Carson City where people buy a t-shirt to let the neighbors know where they've been. It's a Carnal Disneyworld where after your ride, you exit through the giftshop. Unlike a strip club, there's no harsh rules enforced on the wall. Nearly any pleasure can be negotiated. It's like a world outside the norm that's been inflicted upon us by puritanical media empires. Maybe it was the elevation, lack of sleep and a steady diet of Jack and Cokes, but things got really like a dream when I heard, "Hey Joe!" I turned around and it was Joey Buttafuoco. The man from the Amy Fisher controversy who has had at least four actors play him (including Kevin Spacey in *American Beauty*). Why does Joey Buttafuoco know my name? It took a second to remember our meeting at the start of the party. Why wouldn't he remember my name since we're both Joes. He was a nice enough guy. He was extremely happy to be there since he had a near death experience last year. Did he really survive? It was hard to tell since Dennis Hof's birthday felt like an afterlife experience.

There was a Sunday pool party to wrap up the festivities. Since the Party Favors headquarters is on the East Coast, I could only attend the first scheduled hour. When I arrived back at the Bunny Ranch, the place was quiet as a church on Monday morning. Only thing you could hear was Ron Jeremy's snore rattling around the hallways. Everyone was still recovering from the After Party. The pool was empty. The debauchery was taking a break. I wandered back to the lobby to sit on the sofa and wait for my limo ride back to normality. A tired bunny wandered into the room. We started talking a little bit and she fell asleep against me. I was part of "The Pillow Experience." This led me to wonder if I'm supposed to be the one charging? Should I have called Madame Suzette to set the egg timer?

Can it really be another year before Dennis Hof has another birthday? That might be enough time to start my Odious Maximus Hedge Fund.

EPILOGUE

While I didn't do any major interviews with Dennis Hof after his birthday party, we would occasionally swap emails. We discussed a person who was arrested after offering to pay a prostitute with a monkey. The things people did before Bitcoin.

In his final years, Dennis Hof found himself under constant attack from people eager to outlaw prostitution in the counties he had brothels. Besides fighting them in the court of public opinion, Hof twice ran for 36th District seat in the Nevada Assembly. I couldn't cover his political campaign since the Party Favors column didn't want to get too deep into politics. We didn't do a deep interview on his runs. I was also a bit disheartened that he was running as a Republican on his second attempt. Jesse Helms wasn't pro prostitution. When he became the Republican nominee, Hof immediately attracted a crowd I didn't want to promote. He became pals with Roger Stone (pardoned by Trump), Tucker Carlson, ex-sheriff Joe Arpaio (pardoned by Trump) and Grover Norquist. None of these people had ever spoken about legalizing prostitution. These people were empowered by the evangelical crowd that have spent centuries enforcing their puritanical values on America. But these conservatives wanted to pose next to The Pimpmaster General. You might think I'm a hypocrite because I had no problem covering Joey Buttafuoco. But he was a rather contrite man when we met. He had had a near death health experience and mentioned how he'd done a lot of wrong things in his life. You won't hear any of that talk from the conservatives that clung to Hof in 2018. Even the ones that got Presidential Pardons still swear they did nothing wrong.

I had known for a while that Dennis Hof wasn't the healthiest person alive. We spoke about his time getting treatment at the Mayo Clinic. At the birthday party, he was hobbling from his knee replacement surgery. He seemed like a guy who rarely slept between having to wake up early to do East Coast morning radio and staying up late to oversee his Empire that was one quarter of all the Brothels in Nevada. To his already busy schedule, he also lumped on the stress of campaigning for the Nevada Assembly. The morning of October 16, 2018, after his marathon 72nd birthday party; Ron

Jeremy found Dennis Hof's body. He had died at one of his brothels that was a short drive from Las Vegas.

Dennis' death was still a shock. There would be no more emails between us about strange news such as when conservative Republican Congressmen declared a government sponsored Bullet Train would connect Walt Disney World with the BunnyRanch. He wouldn't be calling if a streaming service revived *Cathouse*. We had done our last interview after all those years.

There was one last lesson I learned from Dennis: A few weeks after his funeral, he successfully won his race. He taught me to always run for office in a district so politically divided that people would rather vote for a Dead Brothel Owner than your living opponent.

About the Author

Joseph Corey III lives in Raleigh, North Carolina. He is the author of *Obscuricon's '80s Teen Flick Festival Guidebook, 7 Secrets of Great Walmart People Greeters, Memoir of a Pseudo Killer, Twilight of My Gods*, and *Charles Dickens' A Christmas Carol For Cats and Kittens*. His Five-volume collection of the Complete Party Favors columns are scheduled to come out in the Fall. He has worked on *Candid Camera*, ESPN's *Gaters* and *Danger! Health Films* with the Cowboy from the Village People. He also records as part of the Casino Audiophiles.

Ask him about how he nearly killed the Bishop "Magic" Don Juan in a parking lot.